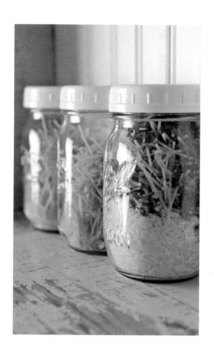

Little House Living

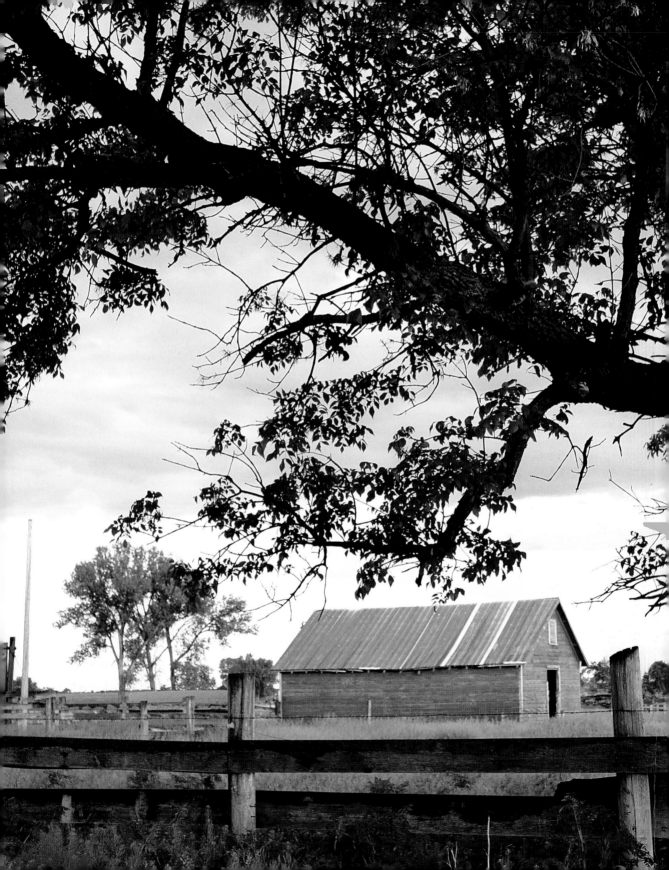

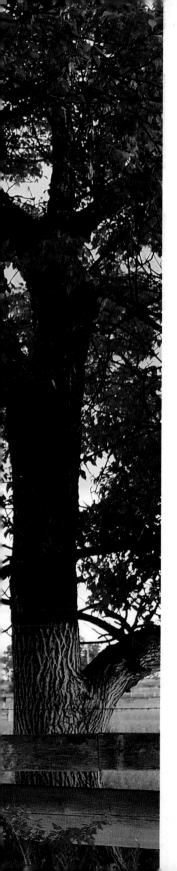

Little House Living

The Make-Your-Own Guide to a

Frugal, Simple, and Self-Sufficient Life

MERISSA A. ALINK

GALLERY BOOKS

NEW YORK   LONDON   TORONTO   SYDNEY   NEW DELHI

G

Gallery Books
An Imprint of Simon & Schuster, Inc.
1230 Avenue of the Americas
New York, NY 10020

First Gallery Books hardcover edition October 2015

GALLERY BOOKS and colophon are registered trademarks of Simon & Schuster, Inc.

For information about special discounts for bulk purchases, please contact Simon & Schuster Special Sales at 1-866-506-1949 or business@simonandschuster.com.

The Simon & Schuster Speakers Bureau can bring authors to your live event. For more information or to book an event, contact the Simon & Schuster Speakers Bureau at 1-866-248-3049 or visit our website at www.simonspeakers.com.

Interior design by Jaime Putorti
Photographs throughout by David and Merissa Alink

Manufactured in the United States of America

10 9 8 7 6 5 4 3 2 1

Library of Congress Cataloging-in-Publication Data

Alink, Merissa.
   Little house living : the make-your-own guide to a frugal, simple, and self-sufficient life / Merissa Alink. — First gallery books hardcover edition.
      pages cm
   1. Home economics. 2. Housekeeping. I. Title.
   TX162.2.A45 2015
   640—dc23
                         2015024538

ISBN 978-1-5011-0426-8
ISBN 978-1-5011-0429-9 (ebook)

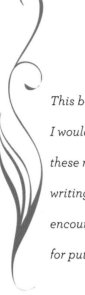

This book is dedicated to my family, without whom I wouldn't have had the drive and passion to create these recipes in the first place. I thought of you while writing each and every page of this book. Thank you for encouraging me over the years to continue writing and for putting up with all of my kitchen experiments.

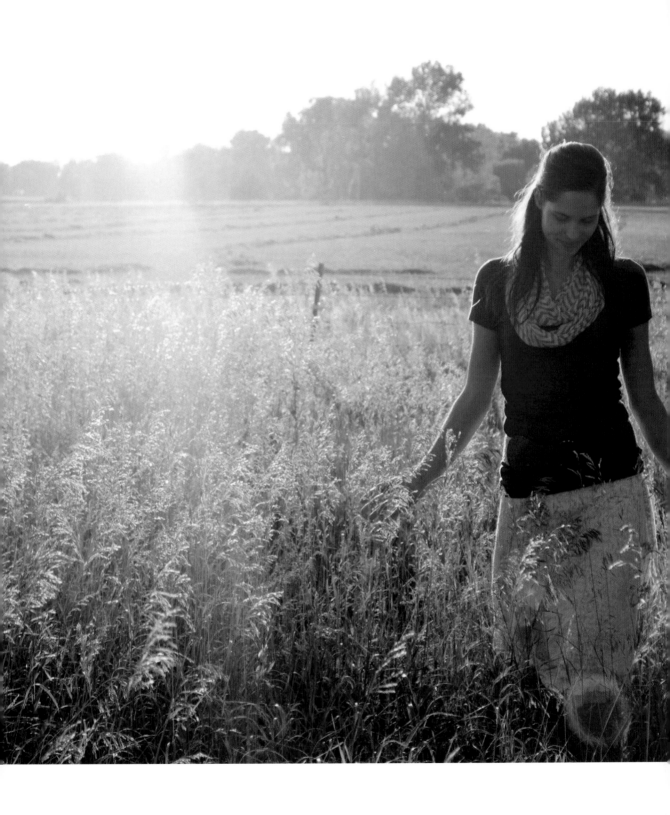

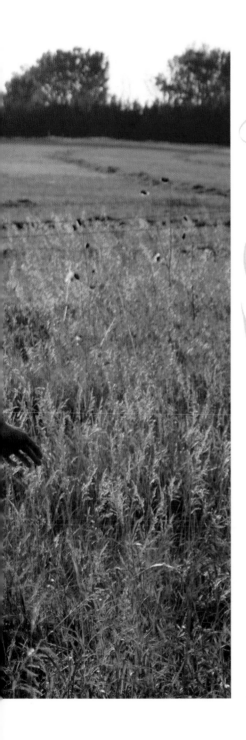

The real things haven't changed. It is

still best to be honest and truthful;

to make the most of what we have;

to be happy with the simple pleasures

and to be cheerful and have courage

when things go wrong.

—Laura Ingalls Wilder

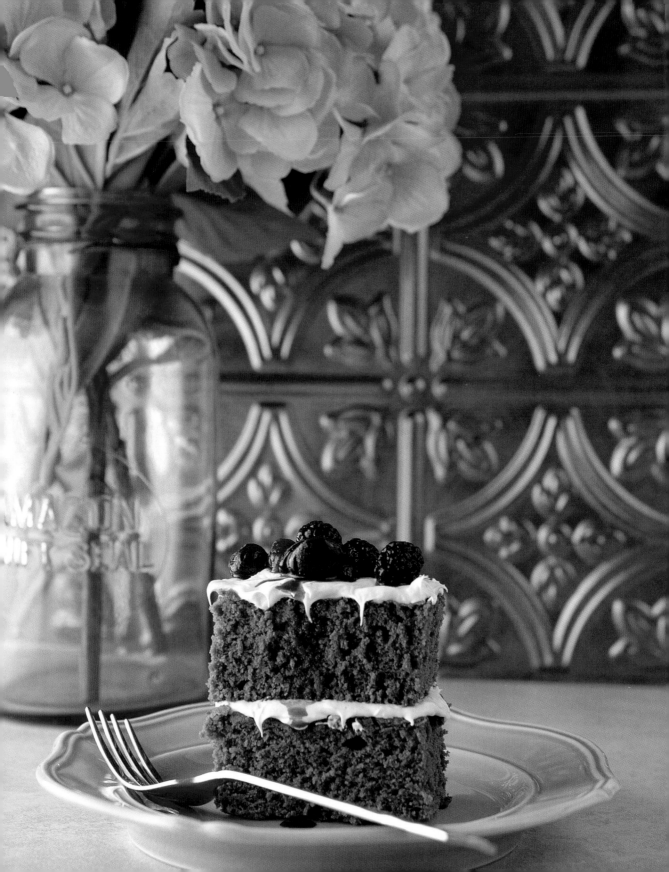

Contents

Children and Pets *127*

Make-Ahead Mixes *161*

Meal Planning with Mixes *245*

Afterword *257*

Appendices *259*

Index *295*

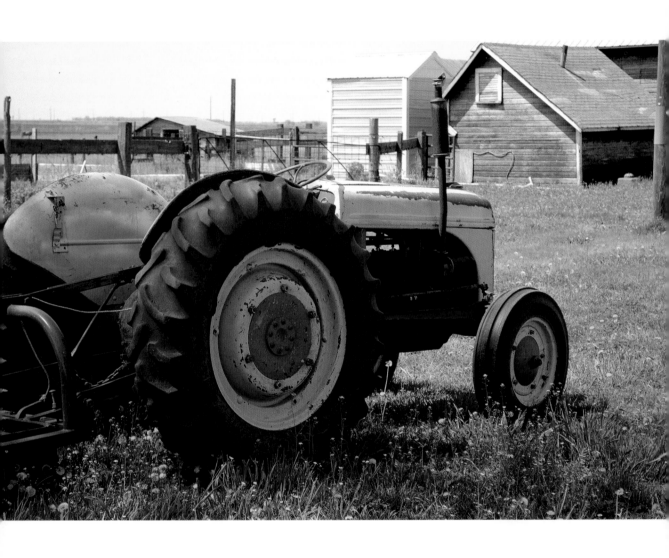

Introduction

My name is Merissa and this is my story. Not long ago I was struggling to make ends meet and barely had a dollar to spare. Living the simple life had always been my dream, but somewhere along the way in my journey the waters were muddied and it was hard to see any light at the end of the tunnel.

I married my best friend at the young age of nineteen, when I still believed that love was all you needed to survive. I'd been a country girl almost my entire life, having the run of eighty acres in rural South Dakota. When I was little I would run through the prairie grasses in my dress-up clothes making little prairie houses and pretending I was living out the life from my favorite childhood book series, Little House on the Prairie. Although my family was blessed in other areas, we weren't always blessed with the newest and best toys, so we made do with what we could find. I had a set of play dishes that my grandpa made me out of wood and pretend hamburgers that he made out of pressed rubber mats. From a young age, what would become my life's motto was instilled in me—I was all about making the most with what I had. Pieces of scrap wood became houses that we built for dolls we made out of sticks; old fence posts made the perfect foundation for a playhouse built out on the prairie. I was happy with my simple childhood. I learned to be creative and my mind was always trying to come up with new ways to play and new things I could create.

Fast-forward to that nineteen-year-old bride. I knew how to be creative; I knew how to cook, clean, keep house, and take care of babies. But what I didn't know was that the next few years would test all of my skills and come close to breaking my resolve.

Right after we married, my husband moved us across the country to Albuquerque for a good job he had lined up. I was ready to make the most of this adventure that I faced, and for a while I spent my first few months of being a wife by teaching myself new recipes that my husband would like and learning how to run and take care of a house-

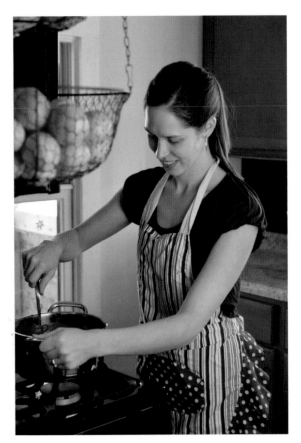

hold on my own. It took me a few weeks to venture out and learn where the grocery stores were and where I could find the best deals on what we needed. I tried to make the best of the situation, but it didn't take long for both of us to realize this wasn't the life for us. The stress of the city had already worn on our nerves and we decided to move back to the small town where we'd met. We packed up the few things we'd already acquired in our married life and we headed north. We soon found a new place to rent and make a fresh start, but instead, things started to go downhill quickly.

We had no money left from the move and in the middle of winter it was difficult to find a job. My husband finally started working part-time in construction, but work was slow since the weather was frigid, and the only thing I'd been able to find was a job delivering newspapers in our neighborhood. Maybe not our dream jobs, but it was something and for that we were grateful. We weren't able to afford luxuries like heating our whole house, so we took blankets and covered doorways to heat only the room we used the most often. Then I got sick . . . really sick. After fighting a fever for a week we decided to scrape together enough money to go to the doctor, who diagnosed me with a severe version of the flu. Over the next few weeks I started to get better, but I never seemed to get back to feeling quite like I had before. During the time I was sick, without the work we'd been doing, any money we had left had run dangerously low. We were able to pay the bills and that was it. There wasn't money left for food or household things. One night I scraped together dinner for us with what was left in the cupboard. I had bread crumbs, orange preserves, and pasta . . . and it was disgusting. I could barely choke it down and my husband, trying not to hurt my feelings, ate a full serving and told me how good it was. But I knew something had to change. This couldn't be what my life had become.

I wasn't feeling good, we had no food, and we could barely pay the bills. I'd been signing up for free samples just so we had shampoo to wash our hair. It wasn't where I wanted to be and I knew it was time to do whatever we had to do to get out of it and put ourselves in a better place.

I was part of a local free-sharing group online and I put out a cry for food or anything that another could spare to help us out. My cry was answered by a kind soul whom I will never forget. She immediately brought us a huge box full of food and other household goods like shampoo, facial tissue, and some other odds and ends. Although I never knew her name, I will be forever grateful to this person who gave us something to help us get on a better path and live a better life, who helped pick us up off the ground and get us back on our feet again. After she left our house, I promised myself that when we were in a better place, I wanted to be that person to help others get back on their feet and try to live the life they really want.

For us, that life we really wanted was the simple life like the one I'd grown up with, and now we were more determined than ever to make it happen. We went from our rental to a camper, to a small acreage, and back to a camper again. All to try to pay off debt and search for the simple lifestyle that we were dreaming of. We didn't have much extra, we paid the bills, and we always seemed to have more month than money.

Plus something still wasn't right. I wasn't feeling well. We ate an average American diet, but I was having issue after issue, from severe stomach pain to a very scary anaphylactic reaction. I tried various types of diets but nothing really seemed to be effective. We finally decided to go to the doctor, who, after hours of testing, diagnosed me with more allergies and intolerances than I can even remember. I was allergic to everything from the food I was eating to the cats living in our house. I remember going home that night and feeling utterly defeated and depressed. My husband and I decided to make a trip to the grocery store to see what I could find to eat and use. I walked around the store and went through all the aisles I was used to shopping in and I just cried. I couldn't live this life anymore, I couldn't eat these things anymore, and if I ever wanted to feel better, many things were going to have to change.

We started making big changes in our lives. The cats moved outside and I started getting pretty crazy about making things from scratch. I'd been making some things before but nothing like what I would have to try now. I started experimenting with everything from making my own hand soap to making my own seasonings. Some of the recipes worked, others failed (some quite miserably!). Everything was a learning experience, and I was bound and determined to still live the best life possible on what we could afford and what I could have.

During this time we suffered losses that we didn't talk about. We'd felt ready for a while to start a little family. But instead of being able to share an exciting announcement with our family and friends, we suffered miscarriage after miscarriage. We saw many doctors and specialists who finally diagnosed me with some further medical conditions. They told us that biological children were very possible for us, but personally, my husband and I had decided the risk was too high for both me and any potential children, and it just didn't feel like the right path for us. We'd already been feeling the urge for several years to become foster parents, and since it didn't seem meant for us to have biological children to care for, maybe we were meant to care for and love foster children instead.

Fast-forward through the next two years . . . we fostered a few children and had been blessed with one little boy we'd welcomed into our home straight from the hospital. We bonded with him in a way that I didn't know was possible . . . to love another human being that much. It was like God took out a piece of my heart and put it in this little boy. He had needs that we never expected or were prepared to deal with, but I spent a great deal of time researching ways to help him. One of his main diagnoses was multiple food and chemical allergies, and for the first time, I felt blessed that I had similar issues and had already been working toward solutions for myself that I could now use for him as well.

After the adoption of our first son, we felt like it was time to move on with life

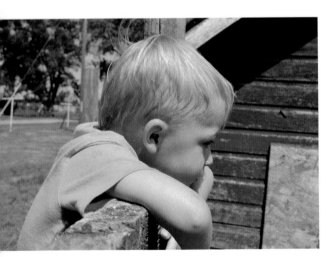

but we weren't quite sure where to go. We listed our house for sale and moved back into a camper once again. When fall came we started to get a bit desperate for a plan. We'd been living in a campground, but most campgrounds in South Dakota close during the winter, so our days were numbered. Unsure of where to turn, we started searching for land to purchase. During these searches we found a little house on a small acreage on the other side of the state. My husband was in love with the little house just from the pictures. I honestly thought it looked like a money pit. But to make him happy I agreed to go take a look at it the next day. We woke up early and drove four hours with our young son to the little farmhouse. As the Realtor showed us around the property, I could barely believe my eyes. It was even worse than the pictures showed, the buildings were crumbling, the house was . . . well, there really weren't words to describe it. The carpet in the living room was three different colors, the kitchen cupboards smelled so terrible that I didn't even want to be in the kitchen, the plaster was falling off the walls, and the ceiling tiles were bowing down with water damage. It was a pretty sad sight. But after we'd finished our tour and I sat in the car getting ready to head back to our camper, I felt this sense of peace come over me. It was as if someone were telling me, "This is it, this

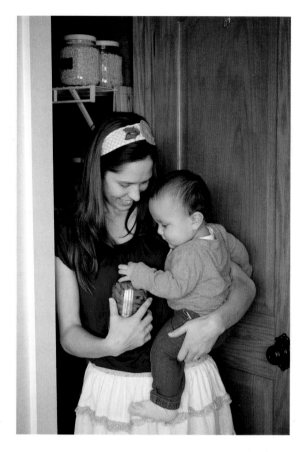

is where you are meant to be. This house is going to bring you back to that lifestyle of simplicity you are still dreaming about." We pulled out onto the interstate and my husband asked me what I thought, and to his shock I told him I felt like this was where we were meant to be, as crazy as it seemed. We called the Realtor back on our way home and made an offer that was accepted later that evening. It was real now, and we'd clearly either both lost our minds or we were following the path that we were meant to be on . . . whether or not anyone else understood that.

After we packed up and moved, we spent five long months renovating the entire little farmhouse from top to bottom, and we couldn't be happier with the results. It's old, it's crooked, but it's going to be around for a long time now and it's our little slice of paradise.

Just a few weeks after we moved into the house we got a surprising phone call on Easter Day. We'd been chosen to be the parents of a brand-new baby boy and he was ready for us to bring him home. We went to him as quickly as we could and just a few days later we became a little family of four.

Since we have moved into the little farmhouse we've gone back even more to a time of simplicity. I was able to keep up with our "from-scratch" lifestyle in the camper even though we had very little space, and now in the farmhouse we really don't have much more space than we had in the camper! I live my life for my family, providing for them in the best way that I know how on the income that we have. We stay creative and inventive because we want to and sometimes we have to. If we feel like playing with bubbles outside one afternoon, it doesn't make much sense for us to drive all the way into town for a bottle of bubbles; instead I always keep my ingredients on hand to make up the things we have a need or a desire for. It doesn't always save time but I know it's better for my children to watch their mama be inventive and rely on what we have, and I hope that one day they will pick up those skills as well.

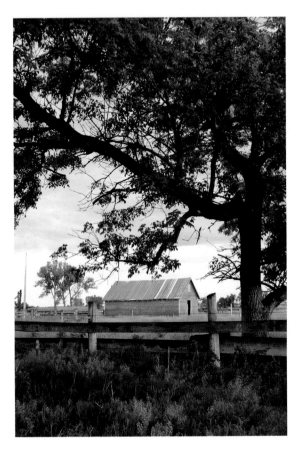

During our last move, I remember going through boxes and boxes of things from the old house. Many of those boxes were filled with notebooks with plans, ideas, recipes, and so much more. As I looked through them while I was unpacking, I felt a mixture of sadness and determination. All my plans for living simply never came to be in our old house for many reasons, but mainly because we just didn't allow ourselves the freedom to have the life we really wanted. We were too connected, too attached, and too busy to let go and live our dream, even though we were so close to being there! I took every single one of those notebooks and threw them in the trash, only keeping the new, clean notebooks. A fresh start. The simple life. We were going to have it at the little farmhouse from now on.

On my walks (which we try to have daily when the weather is above zero!), I pass by old abandoned houses. While I'm walking I sometimes think about the families that lived in them long ago and I think about the family matriarch. Was she resourceful? Was she determined to give her family the best of what she could? When we look at her tools, her daily life resources at the antique store, we might think, "How did she get by using those things and not what we have today?"

She was creative. She was inventive. And she made the most with what she had, no matter what her circumstances were. Instead of spending her hard-earned money on the latest and greatest, she was content with what she had. Modern conveniences were nice but not necessary for her lifestyle.

This is the lifestyle that we live and that we've worked toward for so long. We have more time to spend with our family and more time to create and invent and do the things we love together. We live the life of simplicity that so many dream about but aren't sure how to achieve, and having that dream now has taught us that it can be your lifestyle no matter where you live (whether that be in a city apartment, in a house, or on an acreage), because it's an attitude, not a location.

I'm not in any way a "supermom." There simply aren't enough hours in the day and I prefer not to waste my time trying to be perfect, since I know that it will never happen. I do what I can when my time, budget, and family allow it. Does that mean that I always have homemade laundry detergent on my shelf? Nope! In fact, during the time that we lived in the camper, I simply didn't have the space or place to store homemade laundry detergent or the ingredients for it so I substituted an inexpensive allergen-free version that I purchased from my co-op. That doesn't make me a bad person, it just makes me human. Even if you can only find time and money to make one recipe in this book for now, it's still going to save you money in the long run, and you will have the satisfaction of knowing that you were able to provide a better product for your family because you know exactly what went into that product you made.

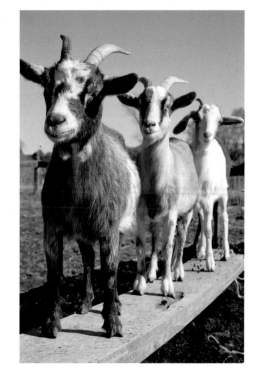

I've always had a drive in my life to help others—

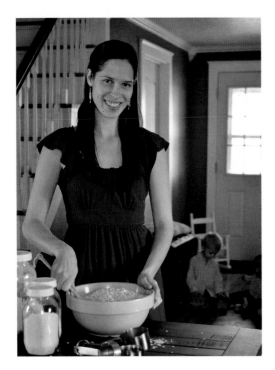

it was somewhat dimmed during my years of distress, but it's always been there. Once we turned our life around and began to understand that happiness is something you choose and not something that just happens to you, my spark was renewed and I've been reminded of my mission to show everyone who will listen that no matter where you are, what your income is, or what your situation is, you can pull yourself back up on your feet as well, and I'm more than happy to be your encouragement and your cheerleader along the way.

I hope this book isn't used just as a guide on what you should do or what you need to do, but rather as an inspiration for your own ideas, a spark for your creative side to help you see solutions to problems in your own life. Maybe you are already using that creativity and making all kinds of wonderful homemade products, and you plan on using the recipes in this book as a supplement to what you are already making. Or perhaps the creative bug is buried deep inside you and by just flipping through this book you are starting to feel the creativeness come bubbling back up again. Either way, I hope you will be inspired to try some of these recipes that have worked for our family. I'm not a perfect person and I don't pretend to be through my writing. Real life happens! We all go through trials in life and it helps tremendously if we can go through them together with one another's encouragement. This book isn't about me. It's about all of us trying to live the best lives we can and provide for our family the best that we can with what we are given in this life. I'm just glad that I can be here with you to help encourage you along the way. I hope that this book and my writing are an encouragement and a light to those of you who are struggling, and will help to show you that you can get through this period in your life. You can create more time for your family. You can create more room in your budget when there seems to be no way. And you can have the best life possible for your family. The simple life that I know you are dreaming of is within reach, and I hope this book will help to give you the push you need to get there.

Getting Started

Ingredients, Budgeting, and Storage

You may take a look through this book and think something like, "Vegetable glycerin? Where on earth do I get that and why would I want to keep it on hand?" This chapter will help answer those questions and help to prepare you for creating a more self-sustainable pantry and cupboard.

Why would I want to make my own/kids'/pets' body/beauty products and mixes at home?

There are a few different reasons why we make our own products instead of buying them at the store. Everyone will have their own reasons and rationale, but here are ours:

1. TO SAVE MONEY. Although the up-front costs of purchasing ingredients may seem like more than you would spend on the products, over time you can see how the costs go down. An example would be . . . homemade shampoo costs about $0.75 to make. A store-bought bottle of shampoo can cost at least $7 if not more, depending on the kind you use. Each bottle of castile soap (which you use to make homemade shampoo) costs around $10 and will make 8 containers of shampoo. Over the lifetime of the bottle of castile soap, you can save $50 by making homemade shampoo versus buying it from the store.

2. SO YOU DON'T HAVE TO RELY ON THE GROCERY STORE. I can't get to the grocery store every day or even every other day. I don't like to spend hours driving to town when I'm out of one item. Instead I fill my pantry and cupboards with the ingredients to make the items I need, and it's really not an overwhelming number of items when you think about it. For example, there are twenty basic ingredients needed to make all twenty-two recipes in the Household section. With just those twenty ingredients, I can make each of the products many times by using the ingredients in several different recipes, not just once. By keeping the ingredients on hand I can always make what I need when I need it.

3. TO KNOW WHAT'S GOING INTO THE PRODUCTS WE ARE PUTTING ON OUR SKIN AND IN OUR BODIES. We want to live the best life we possibly can and that means not adding any additional chemicals or harmful products into our bodies if we can help it. By creating our own products and putting in the ingredients ourselves we can know exactly what is in there and the purpose of each ingredient. Not only does this help reduce our exposure to chemicals and toxins but it can also be extremely beneficial to those of us with allergy issues and sensitive skin issues.

4. TO SAVE TIME. Does it seem like it would take more time to make products than it would just to buy them? In reality, it doesn't. For me, one trip to the store takes about an hour and a half to drive, shop, and get home. And that's if I really hurry! Most of the items in this book take about five to ten minutes to mix up, even the body and beauty recipes! Plus, making the homemade mixes will save you a great deal of time when you are trying to get dinner on the table.

What do I need to get started?

Let's get started by looking over the full list of ingredients that you will need to create the recipes in this book.

BODY AND BEAUTY RECIPES*

Aloe vera gel	Cocoa powder	Mango butter
Arrowroot powder	Coconut oil (extra-virgin	Olive oil
Avocado oil	if possible)	Sea salt
Baking soda	Cornstarch	Shea butter
Bar soap	Epsom salts	Sugar
Beeswax	Essential oils (various)	Vitamin E oil
Bentonite clay	Filtered water	Witch hazel
powder	Grapeseed oil	Zinc oxide powder
Castile soap	Honey	(optional)
Cocoa butter	Lemon juice	

---

* Plus a few more everyday items and essential oils for various scents and variations on the basic recipes.

HOUSEHOLD RECIPES

Baking soda

Bar soap

Beeswax

Black tea

Candle wick

Castile soap

Citric acid

Coconut oil (extra-virgin
  if possible)

Cucumber peelings

Dish soap

Epsom salts

Essential oils (various)

Filtered water

Ground pumice (optional)

Hydrogen peroxide
  (optional)

Olive or vegetable oil

Rubbing alcohol

Sea salt

Soy wax

Toothpaste

Vinegar (white and apple
  cider)

Washing soda

CHILDREN'S AND PETS' RECIPES

Aloe vera gel

Arrowroot powder

Avocado oil

Baking powder

Bar soap

Beeswax

Bentonite clay
  powder

Castile soap

Coconut oil (extra-virgin
  if possible)

Cornstarch

Cream of tartar

Dish soap

Filtered water

Flour

Mango butter

Plaster of Paris

Sea salt

Shea butter

Vegetable glycerin

Vinegar (white and apple
  cider)

Vitamin E oil

Washable paint/food
  coloring

Witch hazel

That's a lot of ingredients that I don't already have . . . Is it going to be worth the cost?

Just about everything you do and create requires some kind of start-up cost. It's the end price, or bottom line, that we really want to look at to determine whether or not making the products will be worth it.

To put those cost fears aside, let me give you another example. Let's say you spend $30 on a pound of beeswax, a pint of coconut oil, and a pound of shea butter. If you used those three items for the sole purpose of making lip balm (which uses 2 table-spoons of each ingredient to create 10 tubes), you could make at least 160 tubes of lip balm. That brings your total cost to about $0.19 per tube, whereas store-bought lip balm costs a minimum of $1.50 for the most basic version, and is exponentially more expensive for natural or organic versions. That's an overall savings of at least 80 percent, but even more important is that you are creating a superior product, and you know exactly what went into it!

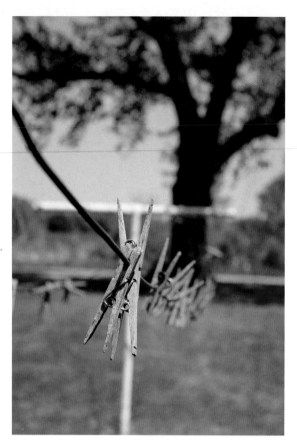

Although the up-front cost of the products may seem a bit overwhelming at first, when you really sit down and add up how much your family could ultimately save in a year, you will be amazed at how much less you will be able to spend on these superb, quality products that are so simple to make. I know that feeling less strain over bills and budgeting is always a good thing, and knowing that I'm giving my family the best I possibly can makes it even better!

But do those pennies saved really add up?

Of course they do! In our example on page 11, you are saving about $1.31 per tube of lip balm. If your family goes through one tube of lip balm per person each month (for a family of four), your cost savings alone on lip balm would be $62.88. Maybe not the biggest area of cost savings, but what could you do with an extra $62.88 instead of spending it on lip balm? Or how about muffins? It costs about $5 to make the homemade Muffin Mix listed in this book. That recipe makes 3 batches of 1 dozen muffins (including add-ins like fruit). Muffins from the store generally cost around $3 for just 4 muffins. If you generally buy one 4-count package of muffins per week, that will cost you $156 per year (and if you have a large family I'm sure you can spend quite a bit more!). To make homemade muffins from the mix in the same yearly quantity, you would spend about $29 per year, which is a savings of $127 per year . . . just on muffins!

What kind of ingredients should I buy? Should everything be organic?

This is a question for you, and your budget. Does it matter to you if all the ingredients are organic? I don't always buy organic products, but I do look for products that are not processed or refined and/or come from a local source that I can trust. Many times you are paying for the organic label when you may be able to find the product at a better price (and the same quality) locally, or just from another trusted source. Do your research and learn about the companies that you are buying from.

What about containers to store all of these homemade products in?

You will need several types of storage containers for the products in this book, such as spray bottles, various sizes of jars, and other containers. You can save money by simply cleaning out jars and containers you already have around your home and reusing them for your homemade products. You can also find inexpensive storage containers at the dollar store and hobby and craft stores.

Where do I buy all these products?

I purchase my products from a variety of sources, most of them online, since we have a limited selection where we live. Amazon sells a wide range of health and beauty products, as well as inexpensive containers to hold items. I love Amazon's quick shipping if I need a product in a hurry. Mountain Rose Herbs is one of my favorite online stores to purchase most of my beauty and body care ingredients. Most of their products are organic and a very fair price. Another large source for us is Azure Standard, a co-op that we order from monthly. They deliver in most US states either by mail or by truck to specified drop sites. I use them for most of my food items. Make sure to check around online for the best prices on ingredients and check local health food stores as well.

How do I know what a good price is for some of these items?

With everything I buy, I make a price list. A price list is a little notebook in which I will write down the last price that I paid for an item and where I got it from. Before I buy an item, I check my book to make sure I'm getting a fair price, and if I find a better deal, I make sure to write that in my book so I know where I can buy the product the next time I need it. If it's an item that goes on sale frequently, I will also write down the lowest sale price that I've seen. That way if I find the item on sale and it matches or goes below the best sale price that I've noted, I can stock up!

How do I create a budget to include some of these new items?

We stock up on various items just about each time we shop and it's a very easy thing to do. Simply add a small amount to your food/household budget each week or month or set aside a small part of the budget and put that toward stocking up on some of these items so you can slowly build up what you need over time. Many items will last a long time depending on what you are using them for, so you won't necessarily need to buy them each month. For example, I only buy beeswax a few times a year because even though I use it in many different products that I make, I only use a very small amount, so a pound will stretch a long way. Even if you can set aside $5 or $10 a week, it will help to build this pantry of ingredients.

Where do I store all of these ingredients and the products after I've made them?

Most of these ingredients need to be stored in a cool, dry place, like a closet or pantry. I personally store my body/household item ingredients in a small linen closet in our bathroom. I place the products inside plastic tubs and containers. The containers are very useful in case anything leaks (and if you have to deal with mouse problems like we do—did you know mice will eat beeswax?). All of my food items for making the edible recipes are stored in my kitchen pantry in half-gallon or gallon jars depending on the ingredient. I love reusing jelly, pint, and quart mason jars as storage containers for many of the smaller ingredients and as containers for the finished mixes

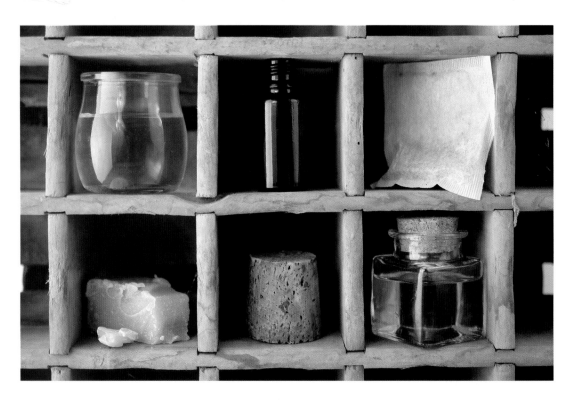

and seasonings. If I don't have much extra space for storing mixes, I will place them in plastic storage bags instead, but I do this rarely as they don't stack or sit on my shelves well, and those pesky mice have a very easy time making a mess of my pantry when I keep things in plastic. If you are dealing with a small amount of storage space, recipes can easily be made as needed as long as you have the basic ingredients on hand.

How much time do I need to set aside to make these items?

As I mentioned earlier, most of the projects in this book can be made in ten minutes or less. I think you'll find it quite incredible how quickly they can be made. Some of the items (like the food recipes) take a little more time to make if you incorporate baking time into your planning. What we've found, and it always amazes me, is that when you live your life in a simpler way overall, even the everyday tasks you do become simpler.

What kind of equipment will I need to make these recipes?

None of the recipes in this book uses special equipment; however, I prefer not to taste wax when I'm eating, so I pick up extra saucepans, spatulas, and other cooking utensils at garage sales and thrift stores and use them specifically for my homemade recipes. Although most of the ingredients won't do you any harm if you eat them, the taste can linger, and something like the taste of beeswax isn't always so nice as extra seasoning, so extra cookware is handy.

I can't use _____ or _____ or _____. If I substitute _____ for _____, will the recipe still work?

Individual allergies can be hard to plan around. The recipes in this book are based on our individual allergies. For more help on substitutions, take a look through the Simple Substitutions appendix on page 259 for ideas on what to use. But remember, there is no way I can possibly test every substitution in every single recipe. A few simple trial-and-error tests should be able to tell you if an ingredient will work or not in a recipe. Be creative and I'm sure you will find the perfect solution that will work for you and your family!

What if I don't feel motivated to make these items?

I recommend experimenting on your own a little. If you aren't feeling creative and inspired, try taking one of your own favorite family recipes and creating a mix from it.

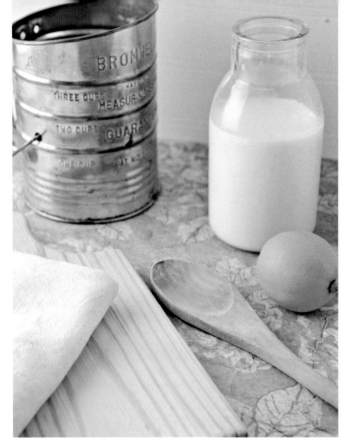

Have a favorite recipe for oatmeal cookies? Combine the dry ingredients and place in a jar together. Now you've got a premade mix that you know your family already loves. You've now become a mix-making creative genius! From personal experience I know that making one mix or one homemade item will inspire you to make even more, so once you've created that initial recipe, take your creative superpower and fill the entire pantry with delicious mixes.

Even better, consider it a challenge to see how many items are in your pantry or in your bathroom that you can replace with homemade items. Don't expect it to happen right away, but evaluate your shelves after a few months to see what has changed.

And if none of those ideas has you feeling motivated, try making some of these things with friends. Have a Lip Balm Party or a Mix Day Party, where you have a few friends come together, bring the ingredients, and create all kinds of amazing products for each other's shelves. If you aren't motivated on your own, sometimes it takes the encouragement of friends to get you started. (Also, when you do it as a group, you can help split the cost of some items!)

Getting Your Family Involved

Instead of letting DIY products and recipes take away from precious family time, it's important to find ways to work together! Not only will your little ones enjoy helping you with your "important projects" but they will also be learning valuable skills and creativity for their future. Here are some thoughts on how to involve your children and your family with these projects.

For Little Ones and Young Children

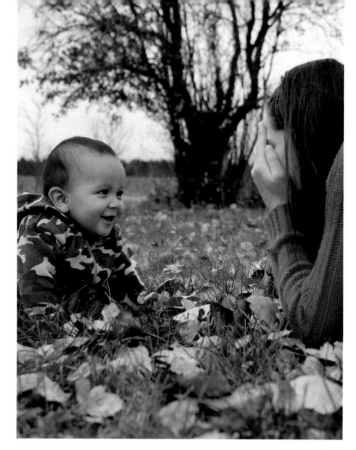

Although it may not always seem like they can help, young children and little ones can be great little helpers in the kitchen and in DIY project creation. Our children are both under the age of five, but I still find ways for them to help me with things. A few things that young children and little ones can help you with: they can pick out the ingredients from your pantry ("Can you help me find the beeswax?"), they can stir the dry mixes together, they can hold the jar or the funnel while you pour in the ingredients, and they can always help with cleanup after the projects are finished.

For Older Children

It's important for older children to learn these DIY skills for themselves to prepare them to live a more self-sufficient lifestyle in the future. I was heavily involved with homemaking projects in my family while I was growing up and I thoroughly believe that is something that has helped me significantly in my life now. A few things that you can do with older children are to have them be completely involved in making the mixes and DIY projects with you and following the instructions, have them plan and make meals with the mixes for the family, and have them try their own substitutions and scents in the DIY and household recipes.

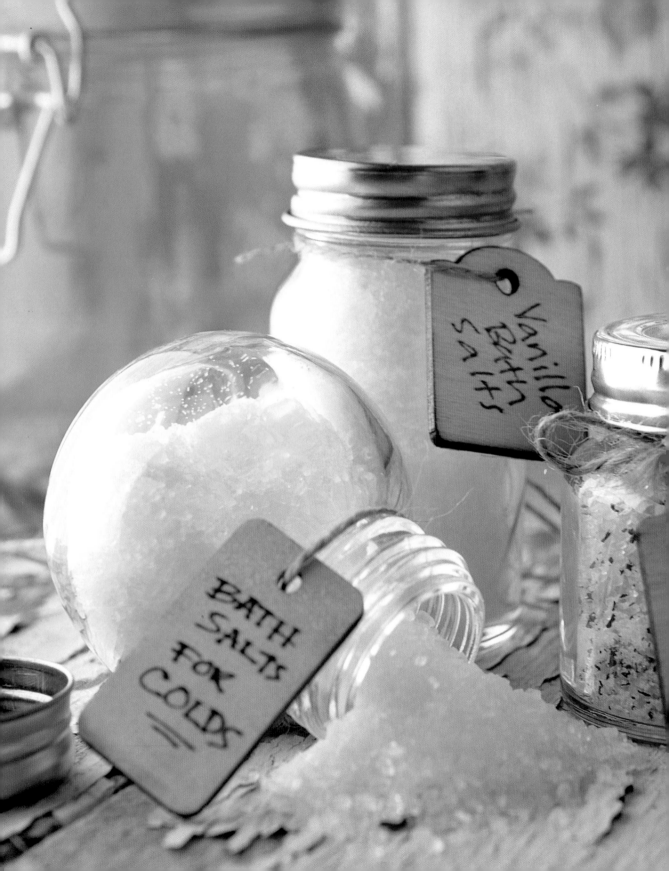

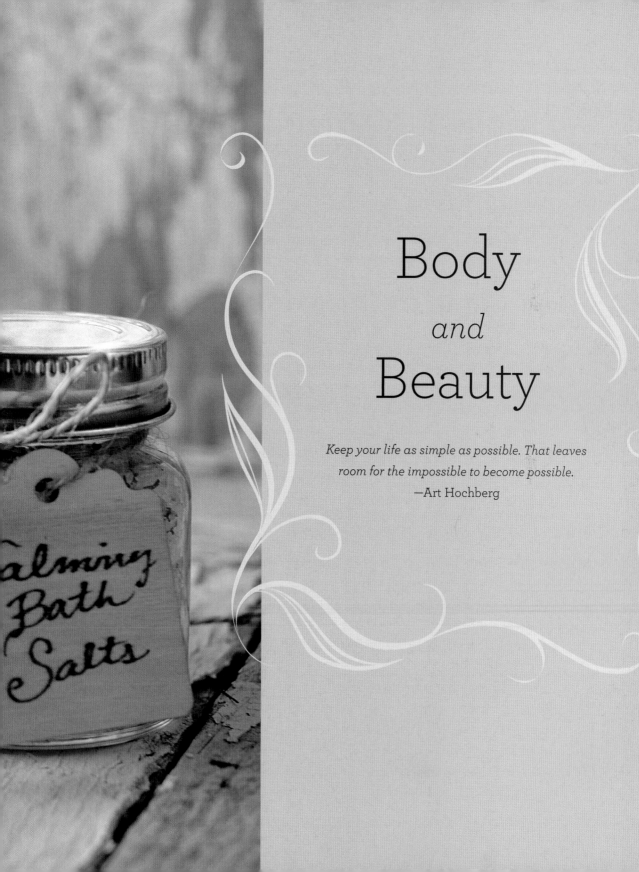

Body
and
Beauty

*Keep your life as simple as possible. That leaves
room for the impossible to become possible.*
—Art Hochberg

I'm a simple gal. After I shower for the day (that is, if I get a shower!) I usually toss on some moisturizer, throw my hair up in a ponytail, and I'm good to go. I've tried wearing makeup and it's just not for me. I guess I figure that if you need me to have makeup on to be around you, then I probably don't really need to be around you. I'm happy with myself just the way I am because, after all, this is the most perfect version of me that there ever will be!

A strong body and beauty routine has never been a part of my daily life, since most days are spent at home at the farmhouse, with only my family and my livestock around. And just so you know, goats don't really care if you look like a mess or if you are wearing designer lotion. They pretty much just want their oats.

Once I started having more and more issues with allergies and intolerances, I noticed quite a bit of drying going on with my skin and I was looking older and a little more wrinkled than I should have in my early twenties. I had major problems with eczema, and everything from my skin on my legs to the hair on my head was dry. In my early days of experimenting with homemade products, I started trying out some homemade body products by making homemade lotion bars. It was instant relief. I would use my lotion bar each and every day (okay, when I remembered!) and I noticed wonderful changes in my skin. Not only was it starting to improve with our less-processed-food diet but the lotion was making my skin healthy and soft once again. From there I branched out to teaching myself to make deliciously scented body scrubs and lotions specifically to help my eczema and went all the way to creating a homemade shampoo that actually worked. There were so many fun body and beauty recipes to create and to try!

Many body and beauty recipes can be made with similar items but using different quantities, which makes them easy to make and buy the ingredients for—because if you already have the ingredients for one, you have most of the ingredients for another. Body and beauty recipes are fun to experiment with and you'll love finding new scents and new combinations that work for your skin. (But of course you will test everything first on a small area of skin to make sure you won't have a reaction to it.)

One of the biggest benefits of creating your own body and beauty recipes from scratch is the huge cost savings for your monthly budget. Why spend over $10 on dry shampoo when you can make it at home for about $0.50?

Not only are body and beauty products much less expensive to make, the home-made versions are also more skin-friendly. You will know exactly what is going into the products and you can simply leave out or substitute ingredients that you can't use. After years of using my own body and beauty products, I've noticed that my skin is healthier, and I have almost no problems with eczema and dry skin, which used to be a huge issue for me. It can be bothersome and rather embarrassing when it's on your skin where anyone can see it. I always personally felt embarrassed because I thought it made it look like I didn't take care of my skin.

I also love giving these homemade products as gifts to friends and family. Depending on what I need the gift for, sometimes one item is perfect; other times, I make several and put them together in a fun "spa day" or "homemade beauty" gift basket. Some great recipes in this chapter for gifts are any of the lip balms or the lip gloss (pages 31–34), any of the bath salts (pages 43–44), Oatmeal Cookie Body Scrub (page 75), Chocolate Body Butter (page 76), and Refreshing Peppermint Foot Lotion (page 78).

There are many recipes in this chapter, so you can always start with your favorite! Or you can jump around in the book and use it as a reference guide by looking for specific ingredients or topics, such as dry skin. If you are feeling overwhelmed by all the things to try, here's a list of the recipes I suggest making first to get you into the swing of things:

Non-Petroleum Jelly (page 28)
Moisturizing Body Wash (page 39)
Foaming Hand Soap (page 53)
Gardener's Healing Hand Scrub (page 50)

Each of those recipes is very simple, requires very few ingredients, and will show you how much fun (and useful!) creating your own homemade products can be.

The Ingredients

There are many different ingredients within this chapter and in the other household and DIY recipes within this book. I selected each ingredient for its specific qualities and properties. Before we get into the recipes, let's take a quick look at the main ingredients you will be using.

ALOE VERA GEL—Aloe vera gel can be antifungal and antibacterial. Aloe vera helps improve circulation so it can help wounds heal faster, tame itching, and heal problem skin.

AVOCADO OIL—Avocado oil is high in monounsaturated fats and vitamin E, which makes it a great moisturizer and gives it restorative properties.

BAKING SODA—Baking soda is a powerful cleaning agent and also can help balance pH.

BEESWAX—Beeswax is anti-inflammatory and antibacterial. It also creates a protective coating to help keep moisture in skin.

BENTONITE CLAY POWDER—Bentonite clay powder is aged volcanic ash. It can be used to absorb toxins while it releases minerals into the skin and gives the cells oxygen.

CASTILE SOAP—Castile soap is a naturally made soap that comes in both liquid and solid forms. Castile soap is a moisturizer and works well for sensitive skin.

COCOA BUTTER—Cocoa butter is high in antioxidants and vitamin E. It is very emollient on skin.

COCONUT OIL—Coconut oil (extra-virgin if possible) is made up of fatty acids, including lauric acid, which is antibacterial, antifungal, and antiviral. Coconut oil is incredibly moisturizing to skin.

CORNSTARCH AND ARROWROOT POWDER—Both these starches have great oil-absorbing qualities, which makes them desirable in many DIY recipes.

EUCALYPTUS ESSENTIAL OIL—Eucalyptus essential oil is an expectorant and is antibacterial, antifungal, antiseptic, and deodorant. Eucalyptus oil should not be used by or on pregnant women.

GINGER ESSENTIAL OIL—Ginger essential oil is antibacterial, anti-inflammatory, antioxidant, and antiseptic. Ginger essential oil can possibly aid with digestive issues.

GRAPEFRUIT ESSENTIAL OIL—Grapefruit essential oil is antibacterial, antidepressant, and antiseptic. Grapefruit essential oil is phototoxic (makes the skin extremely sensitive to sunlight) and should not be used in skin products.

GRAPESEED OIL—Grapeseed oil is anti-inflammatory, antioxidant, antihistamine, and antimicrobial. Grapeseed oil is great for those with sensitive or allergic skin issues.

HONEY—Raw honey is antibacterial and moisturizing. Raw honey should not be confused with regular honey, as regular honey has been processed and does not contain the same properties.

JOJOBA OIL—Jojoba oil has antimicrobial properties plus many other vitamins and minerals that are easily absorbed into skin.

LAVENDER ESSENTIAL OIL—Lavender essential oil has a calming effect and can be used as an antifungal, an antiseptic, and a pain reliever. Caution should be used when using lavender oil on young boys, as it can mimic female hormones.

MANGO BUTTER—Mango butter is a natural emollient that encourages cell regeneration. It contains slightly more fatty acids than cocoa and shea butters so it tends to be a more intense moisturizer.

OLIVE OIL—Besides being great for cooking and baking, olive oil is made up of fatty acids and contains a good amount of vitamins K and E. Because of this, olive oil can be beneficial to dry skin.

PEPPERMINT ESSENTIAL OIL—Peppermint essential oil is analgesic, antibacterial, anti-inflammatory, antifungal, and astringent. Peppermint essential oil should not be used by or on pregnant women or those with epilepsy.

SHEA BUTTER—Shea butter has high levels of natural antioxidants and fatty acids. Because of this, shea butter is very moisturizing in skin products.

SEA SALT—Unprocessed sea salt contains trace minerals that help promote cell health, which in turn helps to promote healing within the skin.

SPEARMINT ESSENTIAL OIL—Spearmint essential oil is not quite as strong as peppermint oil and has anesthetic, antibacterial, anti-inflammatory, and antiseptic properties.

SWEET ORANGE ESSENTIAL OIL—Sweet orange essential oil is anti-inflammatory, antiseptic, and can help fight bacteria. Unlike other citrus-scented essential oils, sweet orange essential oil is not phototoxic.

TEA TREE ESSENTIAL OIL—Tea tree essential oil has antibacterial, antifungal, anti-inflammatory, antiparasitic, and antiviral properties.

WITCH HAZEL—Witch hazel has anti-inflammatory properties, can help in the healing of broken skin, and can help fight bacteria.

VITAMIN E OIL—Vitamin E oil can have an antiaging effect on the skin and will help it retain water and stay hydrated. Vitamin E speeds up the regeneration of skin cells to heal skin faster.

ZINC OXIDE POWDER—Zinc oxide powder contains UV ray protection and can help promote cell health and healing. Caution should be used when adding zinc oxide powder to recipes; be sure to purchase non-nano zinc oxide powder (nanoparticles can be toxic to tissue and cells) and make sure to wear a mask so you don't breathe it in.

Note: Although essential oils can be very useful in many applications and smell great, caution should be used with them. Even though they are a natural product, they are highly concentrated. Essential oils should never be ingested or used undiluted on skin. They should not be used on children under the age of two, and caution should be exercised when using any oils on children under the age of five and pregnant women. Please do research on any essential oils that you plan on using on your skin and always make sure to test any oils (diluted with a carrier oil like coconut oil or olive oil) on a small area of skin first to check for allergic reactions before using it in a homemade body product.

dry shampoo

. . .

If you had told me a few years ago that after I had kids I wouldn't get to shower until after my husband got home from work, I would have laughed at you. I mean, it only takes a few minutes in the morning to jump in the shower and get cleaned up and ready for the day . . . how would adding kids to that routine make any difference?

Oh, the things we say before we become mothers! Not long after we brought our first son home I began to realize the impossibility that was taking a morning shower. If I tried to get up before all other household members, it was too early and I was too sleepy to remember to shampoo my hair while I was in there, or if the baby was still sleeping and I tried to jump in the shower, I would find that it would just wake him up, and of course trying to shower with a little one in the bathroom with you just doesn't work at all and tends to be more hassle than it's worth.

Enter dry shampoo. This useful little product can keep my hair from feeling limp and greasy all day, plus I feel like I at least tried to make myself look presentable. It also can come in handy on a camping trip when a shower isn't available. Grab these few items from your pantry and you are ready to go!

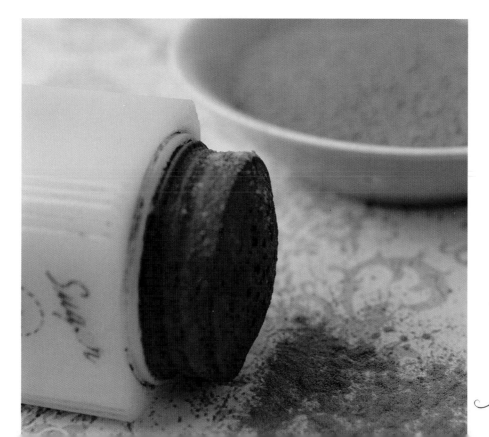

Dry Shampoo for Light Hair	Dry Shampoo for Dark Hair
WHAT YOU NEED	WHAT YOU NEED
½ cup cornstarch	½ cup baking soda
½ cup baking soda	½ cup cocoa powder

Mix together the ingredients needed for your hair color. Place the mixture in some kind of shaker (like an old sugar shaker) or just in a container (you can use a large makeup brush to apply). Sprinkle or brush into the roots of your hair to use.

You can also add a few drops of essential oils to either mixture to give it a bit of scent. Some great essential oils to try in these recipes:

- Lavender
- Grapefruit
- Spearmint or peppermint
- Sweet orange

If you haven't jumped on the dry shampoo bandwagon yet, here are a few tips to remember.

- Don't use dry shampoo on wet hair. It will end up being a pasty mess!
- Give the shampoo a minute to sit on your hair to soak up the oils before styling.
- Start by adding just a little. You don't want gray hair and you can always add more if needed.

Money-Saving Tip: Buy baking soda, cornstarch, and cocoa powder in bulk. They all have so many different uses that you will easily find ways to use them up!

non-drying hand sanitizer

Yes, I happen to be one of those people who don't mind the dirt and the grime and the grease. It is part of life and it happens! I'm not opposed to my family's being exposed to some things to help build up a healthy immune system; however, I'd rather not bring severe sickness into my home if I can help it.

Hand sanitizer is a great way to keep the bad germs at bay. Unfortunately, commercial hand sanitizer can be very harsh and drying because of the large amount of alcohol in it. This homemade version is easy to mix up and is much more soothing on your hands, while still killing germs.

WHAT YOU NEED

4 tablespoons witch hazel
6 tablespoons aloe vera gel
5 drops tea tree essential oil
5 drops lavender essential oil

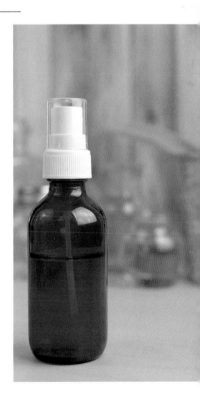

Mix all the ingredients together in a small bowl or container. Store in a small travel-size shampoo bottle or something similar that would make applying easy. I prefer using the travel-size bottles since they close tightly and I can store them in my purse or in my car in the cooler months. (Don't store this in your car in the summer—it might make a mess!)

Tea tree oil and lavender oil are both antibacterial and will help stop germs from spreading. With the addition of the aloe vera gel, this hand sanitizer stays soothing and won't dry out your hands like commercial hand sanitizer. If you still find that it's too drying, you can also carry a small container of homemade lotion to use after applying the sanitizer.

Money-Saving Tip: Instead of purchasing new bottles to store your homemade creations in, simply clean out old bottles from other products you were previously using. Most can be easily refilled over and over again!

non-petroleum jelly

· · ·

Nothing beats the thick, soothing power of petroleum jelly on a patch of extremely dry skin or on a red-from-being-wiped-too-many-times nose. But have you really thought about the product that you are putting on your face? I didn't even give it a second thought until I was told by our doctor to use it on our little one for an ailment. The package says "natural," so it should be okay, right?

Let's just talk for a minute about petroleum jelly and where it comes from. Petroleum jelly is a by-product from refining oil. While there are different grades of petroleum jelly and some can be refined to have the carcinogenic substances removed, it's hard to know which jelly you are buying is safe and which one contains potentially toxic substances.

Furthermore, when you use petroleum jelly, it's not actually healing the dry surfaces but simply creating a water barrier so moisture cannot get into the skin. In other words, it's helping the problem temporarily but not solving it.

Homemade Non-Petroleum Jelly works in a similar way but also provides moisture for the skin to absorb and helps heal the skin. You will still have that instant gratification of soft soothed skin but also the added bonus of healing power. Plus you get to skip all the potential toxic scaries that might be lurking in the commercial product. I don't know about you, but I'd rather be safe than sorry, especially if I plan to use it on my little ones or anywhere near someone's face.

--------- WHAT YOU NEED ---------

1 ounce or ⅛ cup beeswax
1 tablespoon shea butter
½ cup olive oil

In a saucepan on very low heat, melt the beeswax and shea butter. Add the olive oil and mix until combined. Pour into a glass jar or container. Use as needed.

If you happen to have other oils on hand, you could also use almond oil, jojoba oil, avocado oil, or grapeseed oil in place of the olive oil.

Money-Saving Tip: Some of my favorite jars for storing creams are glass mini jelly jars. And there are widemouthed jelly jars for even easier access. Watch for jars at thrift stores or pick up a small case in the canning jars section of the store. They should be less than $1 a jar.

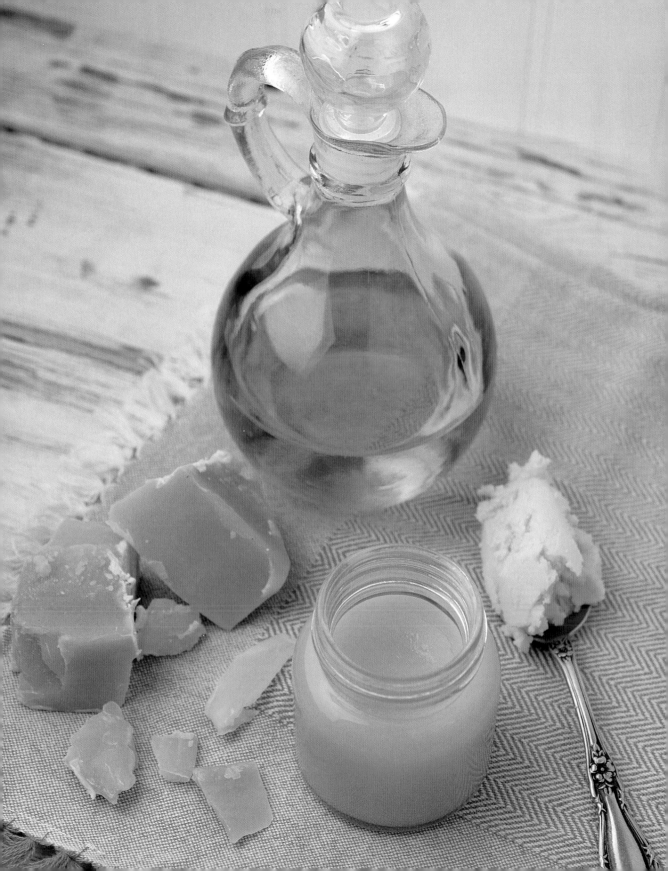

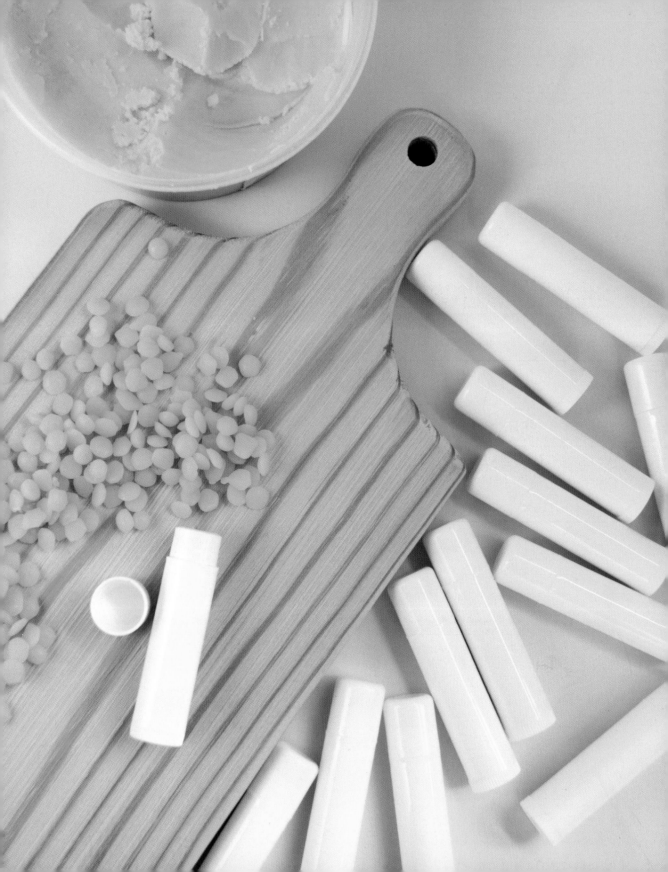

basic soothing lip balm

. . .

Lip balm is one of those products that it seems like most of us have on hand at all times. I usually have a stick of lip balm in my purse, in the car, in the bathroom . . . sometimes I've even found the odd tube in the kitchen! It's something that gets daily use and just about every member of our family uses it. But with a price tag of over $1.50 per tube or over $3 per tube for organic and natural varieties, if you use lip balm all the time, it can start to dig into your budget, especially if you are like me and tend to have a hard time keeping track of those little tubes!

Homemade lip balm is incredibly easy to make, and there are many great additions for it so it can be made appropriate for various situations. You can make a fragrance-free lip balm (using scentless expeller-pressed coconut oil), for women or men who need or prefer a fragrance-free version. You can add essential oils to make a healing lip balm, perfect for cracked and dry lips. Or you can add other oils to increase the natural SPF in the lip balm and make it perfect for wearing outdoors in the bright sun. Either way, homemade lip balm is inexpensive and you can make it in just a few minutes.

You can find empty lip balm containers for sale online. Amazon has a particularly large selection, you can get them for only about $0.20 each, and they are reusable. Let the balm harden and use!

Fragrance-Free Lip Balm

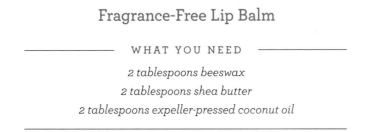

WHAT YOU NEED

2 tablespoons beeswax

2 tablespoons shea butter

2 tablespoons expeller-pressed coconut oil

In a small saucepan (I use one just for making beauty products, not my everyday cooking saucepans!) on low heat, mix and stir all the ingredients until melted together. Use an eyedropper or a medicine dropper to add the mixture into empty lip balm containers.

Healing Lip Balm

WHAT YOU NEED

2 tablespoons beeswax
2 tablespoons shea butter
2 tablespoons coconut oil (extra-virgin if possible)
3 drops vitamin E oil
5 drops lavender essential oil
5 drops tea tree essential oil

In a small saucepan on low heat, mix all the ingredients together. Use an eyedropper to add the mixture to your empty lip balm containers. Let the mixture harden and use as needed.

SPF Lip Balm

WHAT YOU NEED

2 tablespoons beeswax
2 tablespoons shea butter
2 tablespoons coconut oil (extra-virgin if possible)
10 drops carrot seed or raspberry seed oil

In a small saucepan on low heat, mix all the ingredients together. Use an eyedropper to add the mixture to your empty lip balm containers. Let the mixture harden and use as needed. Carrot seed oil and raspberry seed oil have a natural SPF of at least 30. Each of these recipes will fill roughly 10 lip balm containers.

Money-Saving Tip: If you don't want to buy new lip balm containers, you might have some around your home you can clean out. Each time you finish a tube or a container of lip balm from the store, clean out the container and save it until you have several to make one of the above recipes. To clean out an empty tube, simply use the smaller brush on a baby bottle cleaner brush. This will work for cleaning out empty deodorant tubes or shampoo bottles as well.

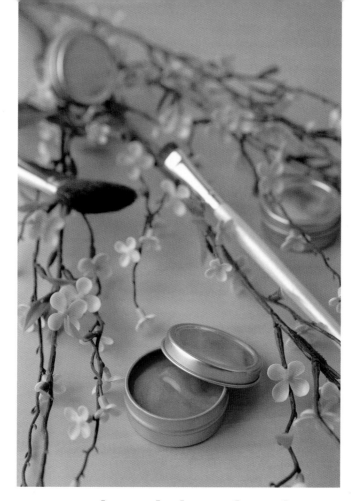

smooth and shiny lip gloss

· · ·

Since we moved we haven't had much time for "date night." It's hard to find some-one to babysit who understands the special chemical and food needs of our little ones, so our date nights usually consist of staying in instead of going out. Of course, this doesn't bother me; any extra time I get to spend with my hubby is a good date for me!

Often we stroll around the yard and the pasture and dream up new plans and ideas together for our little farm and our future. It gives us time to think, a breath of fresh air, and time to be alone together. If that's not a date night, I'm not sure what is!

Most of the time a good lip balm is all I need, but if I want to be a little more "fancy" I will make up some simple colored lip gloss for the occasion.

Lip Gloss

———————— WHAT YOU NEED ————————

2 tablespoons homemade Non-Petroleum Jelly (page 28)
1 tablespoon coconut oil (extra-virgin if possible)
Cocoa powder, beet powder, or peppermint essential oil (optional)

In a saucepan on low heat, melt the Non-Petroleum Jelly with the coconut oil. Add ¼ to 1 teaspoon (depending on how dark a shade you want) of cocoa powder (for a brown tint) or beet powder (for a pink tint) and/or a few drops of peppermint essential oil (for added scent and a slightly "plumped" look). Pour the mixture into a shallow container or tin and use when needed.

Money-Saving Tip: Beet powder can be hard to find if you don't have a health food store nearby. You can always order it online or you can make your own! Simply peel and slice beets thin. Dry in the oven at a very low temp (150 to 170 degrees) or in a food dehydrator until completely dried. After they've cooled, whiz in a food processor or crush the dried beets with a mortar and pestle to make a powder that you can add to homemade makeup!

shampoo and conditioner

· · ·

Making your own shampoo and conditioner seems basic enough until you actually start looking into it. Hair needs to retain a proper pH balance to stay healthy and not get oily or dry and brittle. When creating a homemade shampoo, there can be a fine line between what works for you and what doesn't.

For a while I gave the "no poo" method a try. If you haven't heard of it, that's where you don't shampoo your hair at all and just wash with water. I gave it a good try but ultimately I just ended up with oily, limp hair. It was not a pretty sight!

The best way to get the perfect homemade shampoo is to experiment with different amounts of ingredients and various washing styles to see what will work for your hair. Below you will find basic recipes for homemade shampoo and conditioner, which work on my average, somewhat fine hair. Experiment with the amounts of ingredients in this shampoo and the various types of herbs to create a shampoo that is perfect for your hair type. Make sure to test on dyed hair before using.

Unlike many homemade shampoos, this can be stored right in the shower instead of keeping it in the fridge (unless it's herbally infused).

Shampoo

—————————— WHAT YOU NEED ——————————

½ cup castile soap

½ teaspoon vitamin E oil

½ cup filtered water

1 teaspoon coconut oil (optional)

1 teaspoon aloe vera gel (optional)

Tea tree essential oil, grapefruit essential oil, dried herbs (optional)

In a small bowl, mix together the castile soap, the vitamin E oil, and the water. If your hair tends to be on the drier side, you may also want to add a teaspoon of coconut oil (melted) or aloe vera gel. Add essential oils for scent or leave them out for a fragrance-free shampoo. You can also get prescented castile oils (peppermint, citrus, etc.) if you want scent but don't want to use essential oils. If you really want a natural herb-infused shampoo, add the homemade herbal infusion on page 36.

Herbal Infusion

Add a pinch or two of fresh or dried herbs of your choice to ¾ cup of filtered water and let the mixture steep in a saucepan over low heat for about 30 minutes. Remove from heat and strain the herbs out of the water. Use the mixture in place of the water in the shampoo recipe above. If you've chosen to add an herbal infusion to your shampoo, make sure to store it in the fridge between uses, as the herbs tend to make the shampoo go bad more quickly.

Some herbs to use are chamomile (great for light hair), rosemary (great for brown hair), and hibiscus (great for red hair). Other herbs to try in an infusion are mint, sage, lavender, and basil. Peppermint is a very useful herb to help with oily or dandruff-prone hair.

Conditioner

WHAT YOU NEED

½ cup coconut oil (extra-virgin if possible)
2 tablespoons olive oil
1 teaspoon vitamin E oil

Melt the coconut oil and mix well with the olive oil and vitamin E. If you keep the mixture in a warm area, it might remain melted, so you can either store in the fridge to harden up or just use in the melted state. It will work the same either way. To use, only place a very small amount on your fingertips and rub into the ends of your hair, working your way toward your scalp without reaching the scalp. If you use too much, your hair may become greasy.

Rinse

To manage the pH balance of your hair, you will also want to do a cleansing rinse at least once a week instead of using conditioner. Simply mix 1 part apple cider vinegar and 2 parts filtered water. Pour over hair after shampooing and rinsing out. The vinegar scent will dissipate after a few minutes of rinsing and you will be left with soft, shiny hair. This rinse will also help with any dandruff buildup on the scalp. Since the rinse softens your hair, there's no need to follow with a conditioner unless you really want to.

With my homemade shampoo and conditioner, what I've found works best for me is the recipe above, every other day. You may need to use it each day or maybe even just a few times a week, depending on your hair. If you shampoo and condition your hair and find it a little greasy once it's dried, you can always follow up by using some homemade Dry Shampoo (page 25) to soak up the oils.

Money-Saving Tip: For an herbal infusion, you can either buy dried herbs or make your own! Pick up a packet of lavender, mint, or other herbal seeds in the spring and plant in a small flower bed or container. Once the plant is grown, harvest the flowers or leaves (depending on the herb) and lay in a warm sunny place to dry well. Once dried, place the herbs in a glass jar and store in a cool dark place (such as a pantry) until ready to use.

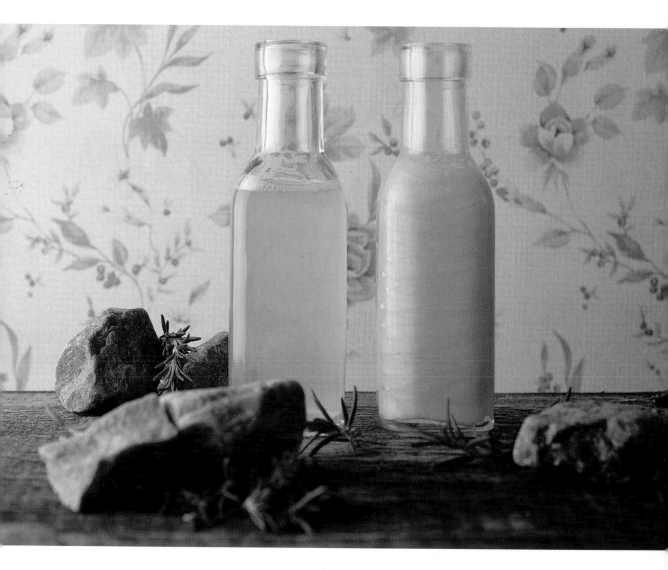

hair detangling spray

· · ·

I usually have long hair (until I feel the urge to cut it) and it tends to tangle quite easily, thanks to the never-ending South Dakota wind out here on the prairie. Some days, after being outside feeding the animals or working in the garden, I come back in the house looking like I just survived a tornado. Thankfully I keep some Hair Detangling Spray on hand and can fix this issue when I'd rather not be sporting the wind-blown look. On days when I'm using my homemade shampoo and conditioner with the rinse, I don't need a detangling spray, but on the days without the rinse, it sometimes becomes necessary.

This spray also works well for my little toddler, who sometimes has a lovely little "rooster tail" on the top of his head when his mama doesn't cut his hair right (or rather, when he won't sit still for a proper haircut).

If you are already making homemade shampoo and conditioner, this detangling spray is super easy to make. Otherwise you should be able to use any other conditioner.

WHAT YOU NEED

¾ cup filtered water
¼ cup homemade Conditioner (page 36)

Pour the water and the conditioner into a small spray bottle and shake well to mix. Shake before using and spray a small amount on wet hair to detangle as you are brushing.

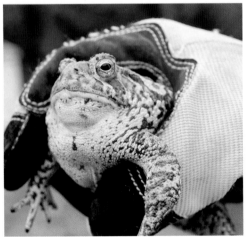

Money-Saving Tip: Save money by learning how to cut your family's hair. Search online for tutorial videos to learn how. It's much simpler than you would think and can save your family hundreds of dollars per year!

moisturizing body wash

· · ·

I usually emerge from winter looking something like a creature from a fairy tale. No, not a fairy or some other beautiful creature—I would describe it more as a furry crocodile.

My scaly and scratchy skin looks readier to sand down a piece of wood than to look nice under a cute skirt. This is the time of year when I whip up my ultra-moisturizing body wash. The benefits of this product last in between uses so even if you do not have the chance to use it each day, your skin will still be soft and smooth.

Basic Body Wash

WHAT YOU NEED

¾ cup castile soap
¼ cup honey
1 teaspoon coconut oil (extra-virgin if possible)
½ teaspoon vitamin E oil
Essential oils (optional)

In a small bowl, mix together the castile soap and honey. Melt the coconut oil and add it and the vitamin E oil to the mixture. If you want a fragrance-free version, stop here; otherwise, add a few drops of essential oils for scent. Make sure not to add citrus oils (lime, lemon, grapefruit) to this recipe, as it will make your skin photosensitive (extrasensitive to sunlight). Here are a few great oils to add:

- Lavender
- Ginger
- Spearmint

If you have very dry skin and need an ultra-moisturizing body wash, the recipe below is just for you. With a few tweaks to the basic recipe, you can create one that is even better for sensitive skin in no time. For those with sensitive skin or skin issues, make sure to leave out any added essential oils, as they can just exacerbate your condition.

Dry Skin/Sensitive Skin Body Wash

WHAT YOU NEED

¾ cup castile soap

¼ cup honey

1 teaspoon aloe vera gel

1 teaspoon coconut oil (extra-virgin if possible)

1 teaspoon vitamin E oil

1 teaspoon avocado oil

In a small bowl, mix together the castile soap, honey, and aloe vera gel. Melt the coconut oil and add it in along with the vitamin E oil and avocado oil. Store in the refrigerator and use as needed.

Money-Saving Tip: Empty soap pump jars make great body wash containers when they are cleaned out. The above recipes will also fit in pint-size glass canning jars.

Two-Ingredient Body Wash

Another great basic body wash can be made with just two ingredients. It's not quite as luscious as the body wash above, but it's very frugal and serves its purpose well—it will get you clean! This is a great body wash for men, because while the body wash recipes listed above are more for soothing and moisturizing, this one is better for a more thorough clean.

Take one bar of soap (any bar soap, whatever is your favorite!) and grate it into pieces with an old cheese grater. Using an old stockpot, heat up 1 gallon of filtered water. Add the grated soap and stir the mixture until the soap has melted. Cool and pour into a large container (such as an old vinegar jug or juice container). You can even pick up pumps that will fit on a large vinegar container for easy dispensing.

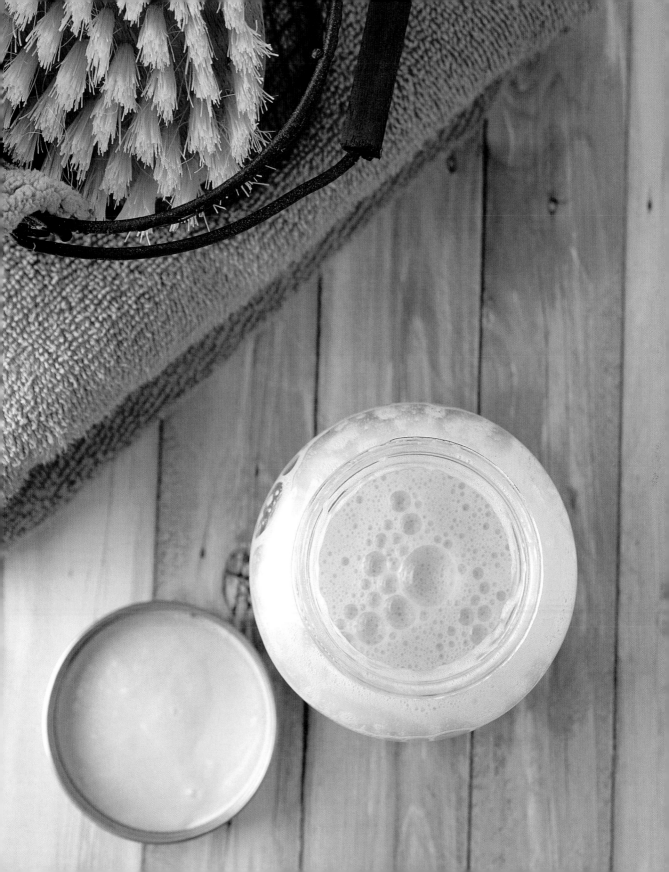

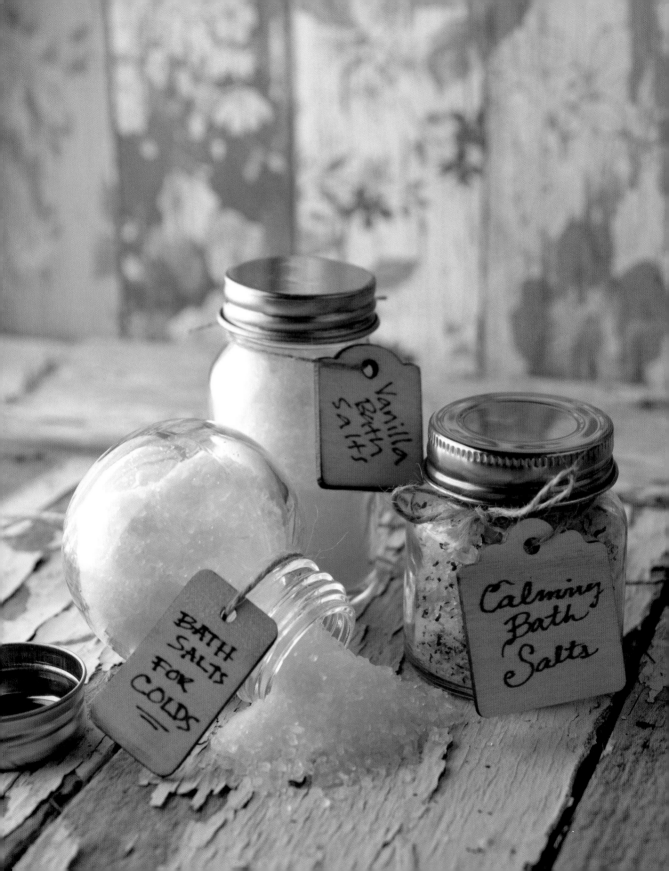

bath salts

· · ·

After a long day of baking or creating new mixes to fill the pantry, I love to relax with a nice warm bath. Creating homemade bath salts take that warm bath up a notch and can help lift my mood and invigorate the senses. Bath salts are fun to put together because there are so many different combos to try.

Besides treating myself by adding these to my bath occasionally, I really love making bath salts as an inexpensive but thoughtful gift. They make a great gift just by themselves, placed in a pretty jar and tied with a ribbon, or you can add them to a larger gift such as a New Mom Gift Basket. (To make that gift basket I like to add bath salts, chocolate, teas, a good book, and a few homemade lotions.)

As with homemade body wash or lotions, make sure you don't include citrus essential oils (lime, lemon, grapefruit) to bath salts—they will make your skin photo-sensitive (sensitive to light and the sun). However, you *can* add actual citrus. Below you will find several great variations of bath salts to try. Have fun experimenting with your own scent combinations to see what you like the best!

Each of these mixtures simply needs to be mixed together and placed in the jar or container of your choice. Each recipe makes roughly 8 ounces of bath salts. Epsom salts are easy to find; you can pick them up at most pharmacies or at many retail stores that have a health and beauty section.

Vanilla Bath Salts

—— WHAT YOU NEED ——

½ cup sea salt
½ cup Epsom salts
1 teaspoon vanilla extract

Calming Bath Salts

—— WHAT YOU NEED ——

½ cup sea salt
½ Epsom salts
10 drops lavender essential oil
Contents of 1 green tea bag

Energizing Bath Salts

——— WHAT YOU NEED ———

½ cup sea salt

½ cup Epsom salts

Juice of 1 fresh lemon

5 drops peppermint essential oil

Note: Store this mixture in the fridge when not in use.

Rose Milk Bath Salts

——— WHAT YOU NEED ———

½ cup sea salt

¼ cup Epsom salts

¼ cup powdered milk

⅛ cup dried rose petals, crushed

Bath Salts for Colds

——— WHAT YOU NEED ———

½ cup sea salt

½ cup Epsom salts

5 drops peppermint essential oil

5 drops eucalyptus essential oil

5 drops lavender essential oil

There are many different kinds of sea salts available, from the most affordable (plain sea salt) to Dead Sea salt (great for skin!) or even Himalayan pink salt (very pretty color, especially for the Rose Milk Bath Salts). Each one of these can vary your bath salts recipes and turn them into something really unique and special.

Money-Saving Tip: Any kind of salt is much more affordable when purchased in bulk. If you plan on making several homemade items, this is the way to go.

hair spray

. . .

If the idea of hair spray brings up a picture of a cloudy room with hair as high as heaven, this recipe might not be for you. If you are looking for something that will keep your style in place to at least make it through the day, you've found the right recipe.

It's a rare day if you catch me with my hair in any other style than a ponytail or just hanging down (because I just gave up and let it be!). With our move across the state I went from the land of dry heat to the humid sauna side of South Dakota and my hair has really changed. Instead of straight hair I've ended up with this mess of frizzy waves. Pair it with the wind-blown look and it's really *really* not attractive! Most days I just don't care because, quite honestly, the goats don't mind the frizz. But on the days when I actually want to look a little more put together I'm glad for this homemade hair spray. It's so easy and I already have the ingredients in the kitchen. I know the recipe looks a little odd, but it works!

Note: The peppermint essential oil will keep the bees and insects away from your sweet hair!

WHAT YOU NEED

½ cup filtered water

2 teaspoons sugar

2 tablespoons lemon juice

5 drops peppermint essential oil

In a small saucepan, heat the water until boiling. Add the sugar and stir until dissolved. Cool the mixture for about 15 minutes and add the lemon juice and essential oil. Pour into an empty spray bottle and shake before using. Spray the mixture onto your hair and check the hold before spraying more.

Money-Saving Tip: When you find lemons on sale, stock up and juice them. Place the juice in ice cube trays and freeze. Remove the cubes from the trays and store in freezer bags. Pull out a cube or two as needed.

whipped coconut oil lotion

· · ·

When we first started to leave commercially made products behind, one of the first experiments that I did was for a lotion. For some reason I believed that lotion must be a complicated process with many ingredients . . . because that's what the bottles from the store had—many ingredients. Oh, sometimes I love it when I'm wrong! This homemade lotion is also significantly cheaper than any store-bought variety. At only about $3 or less per homemade jar (and a little goes a long way!), you can save several dollars each time you make your own lotion instead of buying it from the store.

This rich lotion needs only two ingredients and it's so easy to make! I call this my "winter lotion" because without a stabilizer it will melt in temps higher than 75 degrees. If this happens you can simply re-whip the mixture when it firms up again, or you can use a different lotion formulation in the summer months that is more stable. For summer we prefer to use our homemade Lotion Bars (page 63) because they have other ingredients that make them stay solid.

This lotion has a variety of uses such as a simple leave-in hair conditioner, an after-shave, or even a skin toner. It's a great item to have on your bathroom shelf!

——————————— WHAT YOU NEED ———————————

1 cup coconut oil (extra-virgin if possible)
1 teaspoon vitamin E oil

Place both ingredients in a medium bowl. As mentioned above, your house temp will need to be below 75 degrees for the "whipping" to work. Using an electric hand mixer, whip the ingredients together until the lotion is light and creamy. Place in a jar and use as needed.

Since this lotion is pure oil, it tends to be a bit oily when you use it on your skin. Simply dab off any excess oil with a dry washcloth and you are good to go!

Another great way to use this simple lotion is for a very dry scalp. After wetting your hair in the shower, rub the lotion onto your scalp, not focusing on your hair but just your scalp. Rinse the lotion out of your hair the best you can and follow with your regular shampoo. Your hair will be a little greasy the day you use the lotion but it will improve the dryness of your scalp.

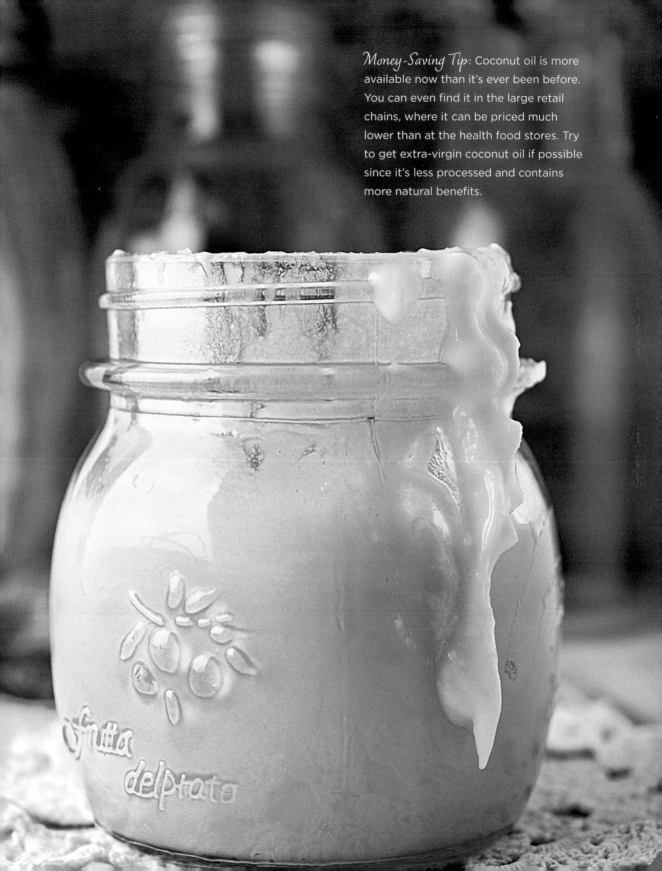

Money-Saving Tip: Coconut oil is more available now than it's ever been before. You can even find it in the large retail chains, where it can be priced much lower than at the health food stores. Try to get extra-virgin coconut oil if possible since it's less processed and contains more natural benefits.

chest rub

. . .

There's nothing worse than watching your little ones suffer from a stuffy nose or cold and not being able to take their distress away. A homemade chest rub can greatly soothe symptoms of colds and flu and can be easily put together with all natural ingredients.

A few notes about this mixture: do not use on children under two, and remove the peppermint oil for children under five. And as with any recipe containing essential oils, test on a small area of skin first to make sure there is no reaction. If you are worried that your little ones might ingest the mixture (if you are placing it under their nose or on their chest), you can put this rub on their feet and cover their feet with socks for the same benefit. (Never ingest essential oils.)

─────────────── WHAT YOU NEED ───────────────

½ cup coconut oil (extra-virgin if possible)
5 drops peppermint essential oil
5 drops eucalyptus essential oil

───

In a small bowl, mix together all the ingredients. Store in a small container or jar and use as needed. Place on chest or feet to help soothe stuffy noses and coughing. You will only need a small amount for this to be effective.

Money-Saving Tip: One of the best and still most frugal things that you can do to help a cold is to make homemade broth. Place a whole chicken in your slow cooker and fill the slow cooker the rest of the way with filtered water. Cook for 8 to 10 hours on the low temp setting. Remove the chicken, take the meat off the bones, and place the carcass back in the slow cooker with the liquid and add a splash of vinegar (you can also add some chopped vegetables for flavor). Cook for another 8 hours and then strain the broth. Use the broth for soups and stews, or drink it plain. Bone broth has been a frugal staple in households for many centuries and contains many healthy vitamins and minerals to get you back on your feet. We store in the freezer any extra broth that we don't use right away.

shaving cream

. . .

Winter is a scary time of year for my legs. When spring comes around, sometimes I'm not sure if a razor will do or if I need to bring out the hedge trimmers. And of course, when you aren't shaving every day, each shave starts to feel like rubbing sandpaper over your legs until they are red and inflamed. Not so much fun.

Not long ago my mom created this amazing recipe for shaving cream. Not only will this recipe help your razor glide along your legs, it will also moisturize and leave your skin feeling silky smooth, so you aren't left with angry red legs under your favorite sundress. And it's so creamy, you'll love using it.

─────── WHAT YOU NEED ───────

½ cup shea butter
½ cup coconut oil (extra-virgin if possible)
10 drops sweet orange essential oil
1 tablespoon aloe vera gel

In a saucepan on low heat, melt the shea butter and the coconut oil together. Remove from heat and pour into a medium bowl. Add the essential oil. Refrigerate the mixture for about 20 minutes or until it has become firm again. Remove from the fridge and add the aloe vera gel. Using an electric hand mixer, beat the mixture until it becomes light and creamy. Store in a small container in the bathroom and use as needed.

Money-Saving Tip: Watch for containers for your homemade goods in unusual places. Hobby stores, retail outlets, and dollar stores often have a good variety of inexpensive jars and containers.

gardener's healing hand scrub

. . .

On our little farm in rural South Dakota, it's important that we spend much of the summer growing as much produce as we can in our garden. Of course, we have the option of buying it from the grocery store, but produce prices here in the winter can really make a dent in one's grocery budget! We prefer to grow what we can for free and preserve it to eat all winter, which helps our grocery budget stay on track. In the Little House on the Prairie books, Pa would say that when they were growing a garden, they would be living like kings. How true that saying is!

Since we spend a good deal of summer in the garden, our hands (and feet!) can get very dirty. And anyone who has kept or worked in a garden knows that "garden goo" isn't always easy to remove. It can be everything from dirt to squished plant juice to plant sap, and it's all messy! After getting tired of trying to scrub it off with plain soap

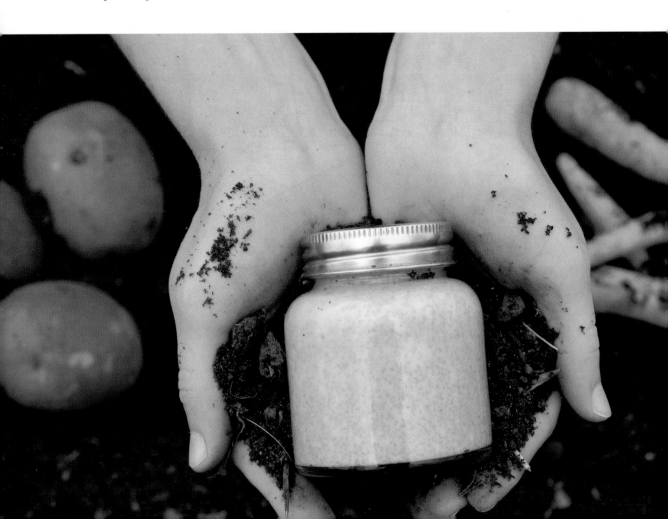

and water, I came up with this simple solution—a hand cleaner just for gardeners. It's easy to make and takes just a few ingredients that are easy to find. Add a bit of essential oil to create a healing scrub that will not only clean your hands but restore them to a healthy state.

WHAT YOU NEED

1 cup sugar (white or brown will work)
1 tablespoon sea salt
½ cup coconut oil (extra-virgin if possible)
5 drops tea tree essential oil

In a medium bowl, mix together the sugar and the salt. In another bowl, melt the coconut oil until it's liquid. (Or you can stick it in the microwave for a few seconds.)

Pour the coconut oil over the sugar mixture and mix all the ingredients together until the sugar is thoroughly coated. Add a few drops of the tea tree essential oil and give the mixture another stir to incorporate it throughout, then pour the scrub into a container or jar that can hold at least 2 cups. Store in your bathroom or wherever you regularly wash your hands after coming in from outside.

The sugar and salt will scrub any garden goo from your hands. The coconut oil helps to rehydrate your hands after you've worked with them and scrubbed them clean, and the tea tree oil is antiseptic, anti-inflammatory, antifungal, antiparasitic, and antimicrobial, so it adds several great properties to the scrub.

Even if you're not a gardener, this hand cleaner makes a great gift for your friends and family who are!

Money-Saving Tip: If you don't have any coconut oil on hand, you can use almost any other kind of oil in this recipe such as olive oil.

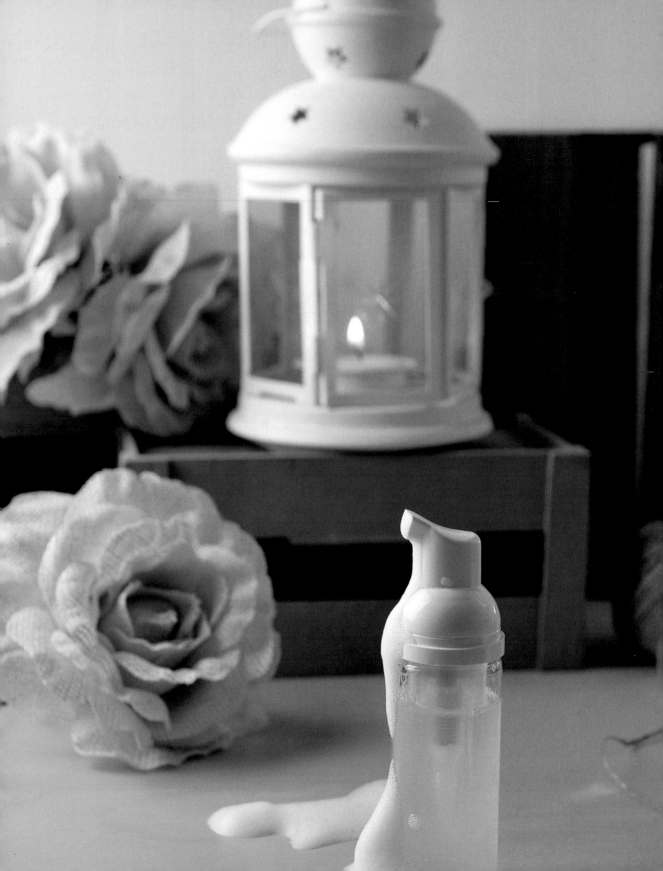

foaming hand soap

· · ·

You know those fancy little containers of foaming hand soap in the specialty stores? I always wanted to have those in my house someday. When I was growing up, a friend that I would often visit always had these in her house and I thought they were so neat and so special. Soap that foams? Amazing!

After I got married and had a house of my own, the reality check came. There was no way I was going to pay $6 or more for a tiny bottle of foaming soap that would get used up very quickly. No thank you, regular soap would work just fine for me. At least until I discovered how simple it is to make your own, not to mention extremely cost-effective. The Basic Foaming Hand Soap recipe below costs less than $0.50 per 8-ounce container.

Just a few minutes and a few ingredients are all you need. Foaming hand soap is really all about the dispenser, so you will also need to find a foaming soap dispenser. You can either reuse one that you already have or purchase them online, and they can be reused over and over again. The recipe below will fill an 8-ounce hand soap container. The basic recipe here is perfect if you have little ones because it does not contain essential oils.

Basic Foaming Hand Soap

──────── WHAT YOU NEED ────────

1 cup filtered water

⅛ cup castile soap

1 teaspoon vegetable glycerin

Place all the ingredients in a foaming hand soap dispenser, shake to mix, and you are good to go!

Of course, you may want to spruce up the basic recipe a little bit, depending on who's using the soap and the time of year. On page 54 are two fun variations to try.

Antibacterial Foaming Hand Soap

1 cup filtered water

⅛ cup castile soap

1 teaspoon vegetable glycerin

7 drops lavender essential oil

7 drops tea tree essential oil

Add all the ingredients to the foaming soap dispenser, shake, and use.

Holiday Spice Foaming Hand Soap

1 cup filtered water

⅛ cup castile soap

1 teaspoon vegetable glycerin

3 drops cinnamon leaf essential oil

3 drops clove essential oil

Add all the ingredients to the foaming soap dispenser, shake, and use.

The antibacterial soap is great for use in bathrooms and we love the spicy scent around the holidays for a little holiday fun!

Money-Saving Tip: If you need a few drops of an essential oil that you don't plan on using often, consider splitting a bottle with a friend or borrowing it.

aftershave lotion

. . .

It wasn't really until after I was married that I found out all the fun little details of my spouse's personal routine. Like the fact that he can't shave without using aftershave that costs $10 per teeny, tiny container.

Deep breaths, we can make it through this! For my husband, the most important factor in his aftershave was that it was designed for sensitive skin. I can handle that! Here's the ultrasoothing recipe we've come up with. Of course, this also works great as an aftershave for women . . . minus the manly essential oils.

--------- WHAT YOU NEED ---------

⅛ cup coconut oil (extra-virgin if possible)

¼ cup shea butter

1 tablespoon aloe vera gel

5 drops clove essential oil and/or bergamot
essential oil (optional)

In a saucepan on low heat, melt the coconut oil and the shea butter together. Remove from heat and pour into a medium bowl. Place the bowl in the fridge for about 15 minutes until the mixture hardens. Using an electric hand mixer, beat the aloe vera into the lotion until the mixture is creamy. Add a few drops of essential oil if desired.

Now you can skip the overpriced bottles of aftershave! This also makes a great gift for a guy who is difficult to shop for; nothing says "I love you" like a bottle that also says "Honey, please shave."

Money-Saving Tip: Extend the life of your disposable razors by sharpening them on denim jeans. Simply push the razor on the denim in the opposite direction from how you shave (if you shave by pulling the razor in a downward motion, push the razor in an upward motion on the jeans) for about 15 strokes. This won't cut up your jeans but it should help extend the life of your blades.

simple sunblock lotion

· · ·

I never knew how irritating sunblock could be for those with sensitive skin until my older son's first summer. We went outside to play in the little kiddie pool that Great-Granny had bought for him and I slathered him up with store sunblock. When we came in from outside I noticed that he was red, but not a sunburn red—a rash red. Not only did his skin rash out from the sunblock lotion but it had an incredible drying effect as well. It was not a good first pool experience like I was hoping for, poor little guy!

So, as usual, we attempted to make our own, and I have to say I'm very happy with the results. Many natural products contain a natural SPF. Put them together and you have a great lotion that not only protects your skin but moisturizes it as well.

Note: Do not use sunblock on babies under six months of age.

--- WHAT YOU NEED ---

½ cup coconut oil (extra-virgin if possible)

¼ cup shea butter

¼ cup beeswax

1 teaspoon carrot seed or raspberry seed oil

½ teaspoon vitamin E oil

2 teaspoons zinc oxide powder (optional; see note)

Note: If you choose to use zinc oxide powder in this lotion recipe, make sure that you do not breathe in any of the powder. And always use non-nano zinc oxide powder, because nanoparticles can be toxic to both tissue and cells.

In a saucepan on low heat, melt the coconut oil, shea butter, and beeswax together. Stir well. Remove from heat and add the carrot seed or raspberry seed oil and the vitamin E oil. Stir in the zinc oxide powder if using and mix well. Pour the mixture into a medium bowl and place in the fridge for about 20 minutes or until hardened. Remove from the fridge and whip until creamy with an electric hand mixer. Store in a small jar and use as needed.

Many natural ingredients have their own SPF (sun protection factor). SPF 20 blocks about 94 percent of harmful UV rays, SPF 40 blocks 98 percent.

Here's the natural SPF of the ingredients in my sunblock. (Vitamin E oil and bees-

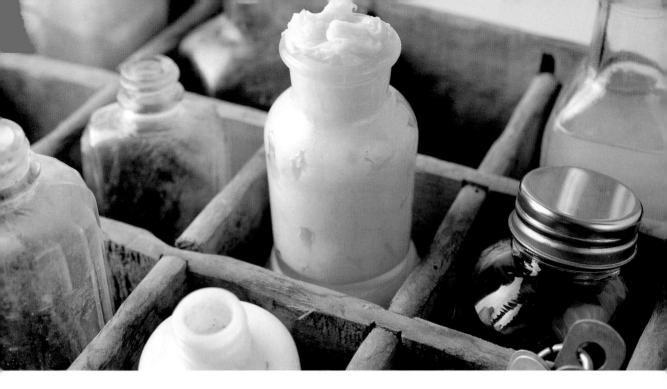

wax do not add SPF properties to the lotion, but both will help moisturize skin and vitamin E will add helpful antioxidants.)

- Coconut oil—4 to 6 SPF
- Shea butter—4 to 6 SPF
- Carrot seed oil—38 to 40 SPF
- Raspberry seed oil—28 to 50 SPF
- Zinc oxide powder—20 SPF

If you have sensitive skin and find that you still react to this sunblock, leave out the zinc oxide powder. The carrot seed or raspberry seed oil should provide an adequate amount of sunblock protection. As with any sunblock, make sure to reapply every few hours as needed or after being in the water. Also, if you are having trouble with the sunblock absorbing in your skin or leaving your skin white, leave out the zinc oxide powder.

If you'd rather have this lotion in a bar form, you can double the amount of beeswax used and pour it into a soap bar mold or into an empty deodorant container for an easy application.

Money-Saving Tip: Both carrot seed and raspberry seed oils can be expensive. Share the cost by splitting a bottle with a friend or two who also want to make sunblock.

sunburn relief cream

. . .

It happens. Sometimes, no matter how hard you try, a sunburn is bound to show up sooner or later on someone in the family. For me this tends to occur in the beginning of summer, when I haven't gotten into our summer routine yet, and we go fishing and I forget to bring the sunblock along *and* don't even realize it until the headache starts and I discover a bright red patch over my neck and shoulders. I'm not good at everything, but with natural red in my hair, I'm very good at getting a sunburn.

My first line of defense with any sunburn is coating it with coconut oil as soon as I am near some (and I usually carry some in my purse). Once I'm at home I will then soak a washcloth in a mixture made of half apple cider vinegar and half filtered water and place the cloth over the burn. It doesn't smell very nice and it won't make you any friends for the evening but it sure takes the sting away! Make sure to skip the essential oils in this recipe if you are using on children under five.

Then finally I will apply some of this soothing sunburn relief cream to help heal the burn. It's easy to make because it uses the same basic ingredients found in the other recipes throughout this book. Don't you love it when you can make something else out of what you already have? Me too!

WHAT YOU NEED

½ cup coconut oil (extra-virgin if possible)
1 tablespoon aloe vera gel
5 drops peppermint essential oil

Mix the ingredients together in a small bowl. Place in a container and apply to a sunburn as needed.

How does this wonderful cream help your poor burned skin? Well, coconut oil adds antioxidants and moisture back to your skin to help heal the burn. Aloe vera gel contains anti-inflammatory properties that help bring down the swelling and redness. Peppermint essential oil helps cool the stinging burn and soothe any itching. All sunburn-beating powerhouses . . . mix them together and apply liberally and you will feel better by morning!

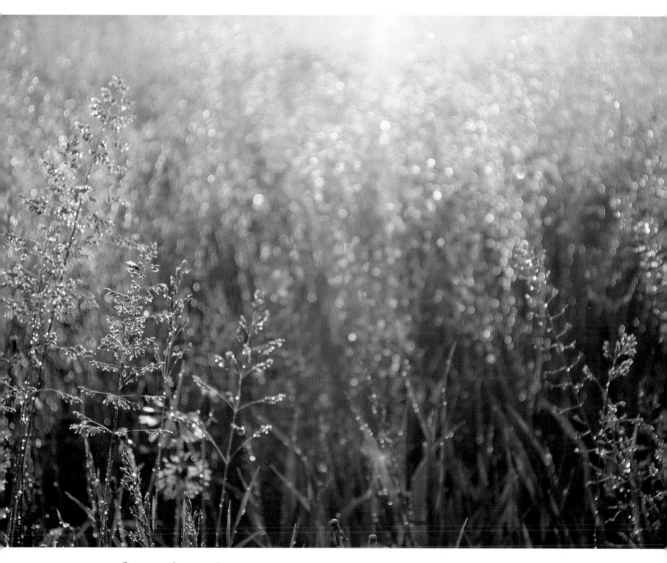

Money-Saving Tip: If you plan on using quite a bit of aloe vera gel in recipes, it might make sense for you to grow your own plant and harvest the gel yourself. Look in the succulents section of your local greenhouse and find a healthy aloe plant. Then, simply cut off a leaf and remove the gel to use as needed. Anything with fresh aloe gel should be stored in the fridge.

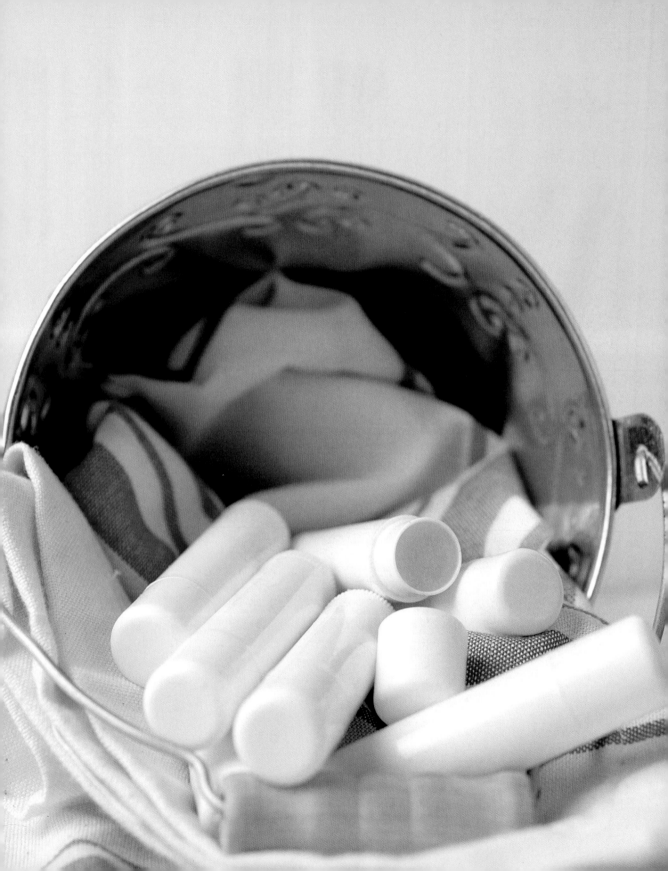

zit zapper sticks

. . .

No one wants to have to deal with acne, at any age. It's embarrassing and can be painful. I wasn't one of those who suffered with acne while I was a teen (my skin was too dry), but I did suffer from it for a while as an adult while I was going through diet changes to discover what my body could and couldn't handle.

During that time I wanted to find a natural cure for my acne that wouldn't dry out my skin or make it feel any worse than it already did. Once I found a good formula, I decided to put it in an empty lip balm tube to make it an easy-to-use Zit Zapper in stick form.

Over the last few years I've changed up my Zit Zapper recipe for different skin types for friends and friends' families to use. You may have to try a few varieties to figure out which one works best for your skin type.

Basic Zit Zapper

——————— WHAT YOU NEED ———————

⅛ cup coconut oil (extra-virgin if possible)
½ teaspoon beeswax
7 drops tea tree essential oil

In a small saucepan on low heat, melt the coconut oil and beeswax together. Remove from heat and add the drops of tea tree oil. Mix and use an eyedropper to fill up empty lip balm tubes for easy application. Spot-treat as needed.

Since they have similar properties, you can also substitute lavender oil for the tea tree oil if you prefer the scent—and it may work better for your skin, depending on your body.

Clay Zit Zapper

——————— WHAT YOU NEED ———————

⅛ cup coconut oil (extra-virgin if possible)
1 teaspoon bentonite clay powder

Warm the coconut oil, then mix the ingredients together in a bowl. Pour the mixture into an empty lip balm container and let it harden. With this version of the Zit Zapper, apply to your face before bed and rinse off in the morning.

Money-Saving Tip: Look for bentonite clay powder in bulk at health food stores. You can usually get it for a better price and just buy the amount you really need.

Facial Washes

Facial washes can be beneficial to those dealing with acne. Here are a few for you to try. Remember, you may have to experiment to see what works best for your skin. If you have very sensitive skin, you may want to stick with the green tea rinse or even plain water.

APPLE CIDER VINEGAR. Create a face wash with 1 part apple cider vinegar to 2 parts filtered water.

BAKING SODA. Create a paste with baking soda and filtered water and apply to your face as needed for spot treatment or over your entire face. Leave on for about 15 minutes and then rinse off.

LEMON JUICE. Squeeze a fresh lemon and apply the juice to your entire face. Leave the juice on for a few minutes before rinsing off.

GREEN TEA. Green tea makes a great face wash because of its antibacterial properties. Brew up a strong pot of tea (stronger than one that you would drink), cool, and use as a face rinse.

WITCH HAZEL. Witch hazel also makes a good astringent. Apply with a washcloth or cotton ball and rinse off with water.

lotion bars

· · ·

Many years ago my mom started making and giving me homemade lotion bars to use instead of commercial lotion. They worked great on my skin, but I really disliked the "bar" style. A traditional lotion bar is made in a soap bar mold and you simply apply the lotion bar like you are using a soap bar on your body. I loved the lotion formula but found that it would melt in my hands, especially in the summer. And maybe it's just me, but I really dislike having lotion on my hands.

For me the solution was simple: I came across some empty deodorant tubes while surfing the Web one day and thought, "Those would be perfect!" Not only would I avoid having slippery hands after applying the lotion, but the lotion would stay easy to apply throughout the year. We especially love using this lotion in the summer because unless it gets really hot, it does not melt.

─────────── WHAT YOU NEED ───────────

1 cup beeswax
¾ cup coconut oil (extra-virgin if possible)
¾ cup shea butter

Place all the ingredients in a medium saucepan over low heat until they have melted and are mixed together.

Have your empty deodorant containers ready and standing upright with the lids off on a piece of waxed paper. Pour the melted lotion mixture into the containers. This recipe will fill 6 empty deodorant containers. Let the full deodorant containers stand at room temperature until the lotion mixture has hardened.

You can, of course, make traditional-style lotion bars by simply pouring your lotion ingredients into a soap mold and letting them harden. Store the lotion bars in small bags until ready to use.

These lotion bars are so simple, with only three ingredients, but the lotion is incredibly moisturizing and works so well. It's a great basic lotion to use any time of year and works great on most types of skin. We also like to use this on mild eczema. Since it's a thicker lotion, it works well for that kind of application, and the antioxidant properties of the coconut oil help heal skin. In our house we all use lotion bars, from the baby to my hubby! It's a basic staple that is always available in our bathroom linen closet.

You can always add a few drops of essential oil into your lotion bar recipe to give it a pleasant scent, or if you leave it as is, it will simply smell faintly of coconut oil. We don't add essential oils to this recipe since we use it on all family members, including the children.

Money-Saving Tip: If you'd rather not purchase empty deodorant containers, simply start saving the ones you are using now. Once they are empty, wash them out well and reuse for homemade lotions and homemade deodorant.

eczema cream

· · ·

When our older son was just two months old, I took him to the doctor about a rash that covered his entire body. We discovered that not only was he suffering from a respiratory infection but he also was having major allergy issues with his food. We began a trial-and-error diet to find him something else to eat. Eventually we found something that worked for him but he still suffered from eczema. The doctor prescribed lotion after lotion and finally prescribed a steroid cream. As she was going through the instructions for application, I remember thinking, "Why is this something that is okay to put on my baby's skin but I need to wash my hands immediately after application?" It didn't sit well with me.

So I started a long search for just the right balance of ingredients for a soothing eczema lotion that would work for him. I knew it needed to be full of natural fatty acids to help heal his skin and be ultra-moisturizing while also being thick enough to stay in place and do its job well. I think, after much trial and error, I've finally found the perfect solution and we've been so happy with the results. As a toddler he still suffers from eczema from time to time (mostly from environmental allergies now), but a few days of applying this sweet cream and he's good to go again. If you have someone in your family who suffers from eczema, I hope you will try this cream and I hope it works for you! There's nothing worse than dealing with the pain and itching of eczema.

───────────── WHAT YOU NEED ─────────────

¼ cup coconut oil (extra-virgin if possible)

2 tablespoons shea butter

1 tablespoon beeswax

1 tablespoon avocado oil

1 tablespoon aloe vera gel

1 teaspoon vitamin E oil

In a saucepan on low heat, melt together the coconut oil, shea butter, and beeswax. Remove from heat and pour into a medium bowl. Mix in the avocado oil, aloe vera gel, and vitamin E oil. Blend well and refrigerate the mixture until it has hardened (about 20 minutes). Using an electric hand mixer, whip the lotion until it becomes light and fluffy. Apply to the skin as needed for treatment of eczema or extremely dry skin.

Money-Saving Tip: When purchasing vitamin E oil, you will save money by buying the liquid version instead of the capsules, plus it's easier to measure for your recipes. Make sure the vitamin E is a nice dark color and doesn't have added ingredients.

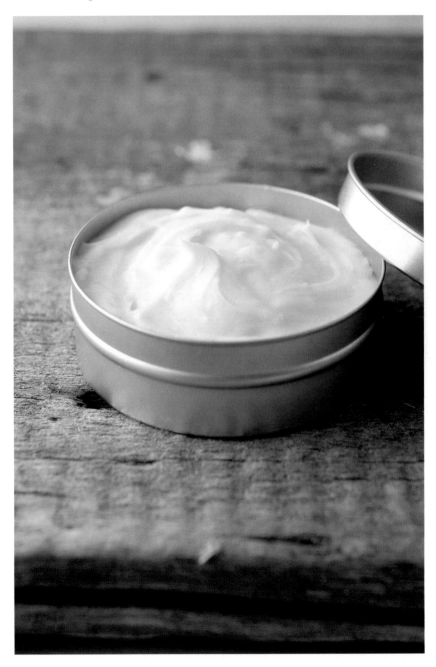

face masks

· · ·

"Girls' night" doesn't happen often in my house full of boys, but when it does it's all about using what we have to make a fun night.

My gal friends and their little girls love my homemade face mask recipes! When we get together we like to make the basic recipes and then add to them for some fun (and sometimes interesting!) combinations. Out of these three recipes, my friends' favorite by far is the Coffee and Cocoa Mask . . . what girl doesn't love that combination? And when you can turn those loves into something that softens and smooths skin? That's a winner in my book!

These three basic face mask recipes use things that you have in the kitchen. Each will help moisturize, rejuvenate, and refresh your skin.

Minty Fresh Face Mask

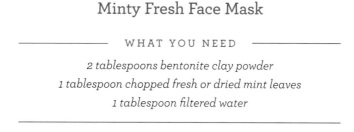

WHAT YOU NEED

2 tablespoons bentonite clay powder
1 tablespoon chopped fresh or dried mint leaves
1 tablespoon filtered water

Mix all the ingredients together and apply gently to face. Let the mask dry and remove by rinsing with water and a wet washcloth.

Oatmeal and Honey Face Mask

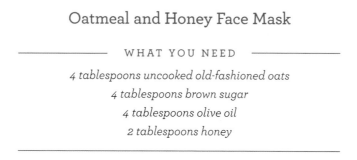

WHAT YOU NEED

4 tablespoons uncooked old-fashioned oats
4 tablespoons brown sugar
4 tablespoons olive oil
2 tablespoons honey

In a blender, blend the oats with the brown sugar until it forms a light powder. Place the brown sugar blend in a small bowl and add the olive oil and honey. Mix all the ingredients together well. Apply to face and leave on until dry. Rinse off gently.

Coffee and Cocoa Face Mask

—————————— WHAT YOU NEED ——————————

4 tablespoons ground or instant coffee
4 tablespoons cocoa powder
4 tablespoons olive oil
2 tablespoons honey

If the coffee isn't finely ground, start by grinding it into a finer powder. Pour into a small bowl and add the cocoa powder, olive oil, and honey. Mix all the ingredients together well. Warm up the entire mixture by heating it in the microwave or by placing the bowl in a larger bowl of warm water. Apply to face by dabbing gently onto skin (do not rub), let it dry on your skin, and gently wash off.

Money-Saving Tip: You can make a face mask with just about anything natural you can find in your kitchen. Experiment with substituting some of the ingredients in the recipes above with other items you have on hand to find more face masks you will love. Avocados make a great base for a face mask, as do pureed pumpkin and egg whites. Dig through your produce drawer and get creative!

healing salve

· · ·

When our older son was just eight months old, I knew something wasn't right. He wasn't trying to crawl like other little ones his age and he hadn't even been able to sit up yet on his own. We connected with an amazing physical therapist that worked her magic over the next eight months on our little boy. We went through everything from special muscle tape to leg braces, and the day when our little boy took his first steps was a miraculous one.

This healing salve is another wonderful recipe from my mom's experiments. When my older son started walking, I gave my mom a call and asked her if she had some kind of first aid cream that I could try. I knew it was inevitable that our little boy was going to suffer his fair share of cuts and bruises and I wanted to be ready—and for good reason: he's now an active little boy!

Once he found the strength to go, he was determined to go and keep going. Now he rarely walks anywhere—he runs, he skips, and he jumps. He's on the move and it's all we can do to try to keep up.

And I was right to be on top of the cuts and bruises. I feel like there is a new one every day! I'm so grateful to Grandma for creating this wonderful recipe.

WHAT YOU NEED

¼ cup grapeseed oil

¼ cup coconut oil
(extra-virgin if possible)

3 tablespoons beeswax

10 drops tea tree essential oil

8 drops lavender essential oil

5 drops lemon essential oil

½ teaspoon vitamin E oil

In a saucepan on low heat, melt together the grapeseed oil, coconut oil, and beeswax. Remove from heat and add the essential oils and the vitamin E oil. Pour into a small container and use on cuts and scratches as needed.

This recipe is a perfect addition to a first aid kit and a good item to take camping. Or, if you are like us, keep it next to the door for whenever someone comes in the house with tears and a new bump.

Money-Saving Tip: Make a good basic first aid kit with Healing Salve, bentonite clay powder, some gauze, and bandages. Just these few items will help solve most ailments. We keep these mini kits in our camper and car.

burn salve

· · ·

We have our fair share of bumps and bruises around our home, and I tend to be particularly accident-prone for some reason.

One afternoon I decided to cook something on the stove in my frying pan. As it started cooking I noticed an odd smell like campfire smoke coming from something. I ran to the windows to check outside and opened the door but I didn't smell anything out of the ordinary. I followed the smell right to my stovetop where I was cooking. But I still couldn't figure it out because my food was not burning. So I turned off the stove and picked up the pan, and on the bottom was a toy that somehow had gotten stuck and was on fire! Not using common sense, I grabbed the burning toy with my bare fingers and tossed it in the sink that was full of water. I felt pretty proud of myself for stopping the fire until my fingers started to ache!

Luckily we have a good homemade burn salve that we keep "on hand" at all times. (And yes, I do keep some in the kitchen now!) This recipe takes only about five minutes to put together and it's incredibly soothing for any minor burns. The raw honey and coconut oil will help along the healing process.

———————————————— WHAT YOU NEED ————————————————

¼ cup raw honey
1 tablespoon coconut oil (extra-virgin if possible)
1 tablespoon aloe vera (gel or liquid)

Mix all the ingredients together. If you don't use this right away and the mixture starts to crystallize, simply place the container or jar in warm water and the honey will go back to its regular texture. Before you use this salve, dab some apple cider vinegar over the burn. This will help restore the natural pH balance of your skin. After you cleanse with vinegar and place the salve on the affected area, you can cover with a Band-Aid or gauze. This salve is for minor burns only; you should seek medical attention for severe burns.

Money-Saving Tip: Ask around your local area to see if anyone sells raw honey. You might be able to find a great deal and support a local business at the same time.

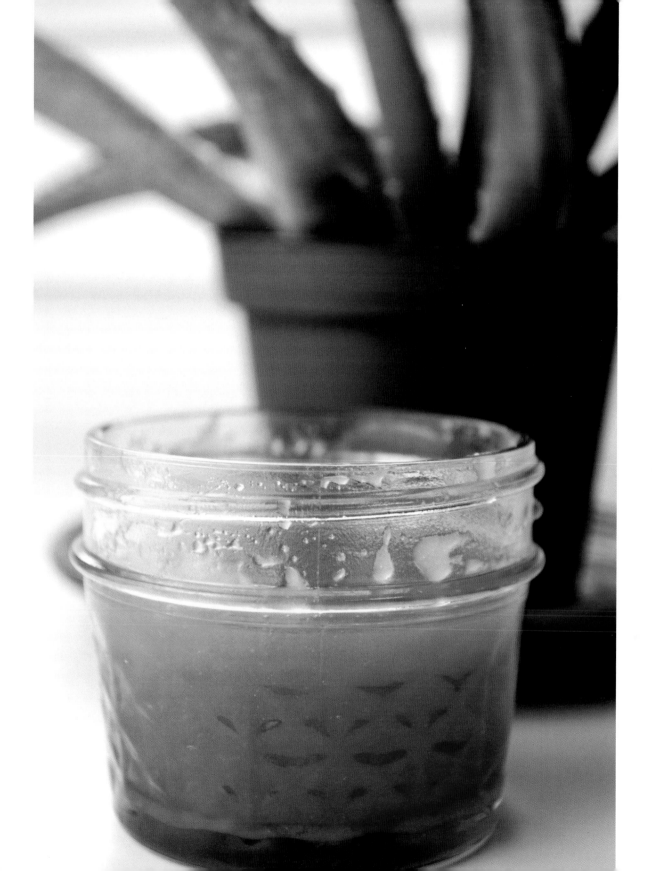

deodorant

. . .

I like to take credit for inspiring my mom to create her own homemade beauty products, but I know I can't since she's been doing it for much longer than I have. I do think, though, that now that we've joined forces in our homemade-everything ways, we've both become more inspired by what the other one can create.

Not long ago I asked her to create a great homemade deodorant that actually worked. I'd attempted it a few times but nothing I used was actually effective, especially not in the summer.

Note: Natural deodorant is a deodorant only, not an antiperspirant. In commercial products, the antiperspirant is created when aluminum is added to the mixture to plug sweat glands. Sweating is natural, but that doesn't mean you have to smell.

WHAT YOU NEED

¼ cup coconut oil (extra-virgin if possible)

¼ cup shea butter

¼ cup beeswax

2 tablespoons bentonite clay powder

2 tablespoons baking soda

2 tablespoons arrowroot powder or cornstarch

5 drops eucalyptus essential oil

5 drops sweet orange essential oil

5 drops rosemary essential oil

8 drops tea tree essential oil

In a saucepan on low heat, melt the coconut oil, shea butter, and beeswax together. Remove from heat and stir in the clay, baking soda, arrowroot powder or cornstarch, and essential oils. Blend well.

Have empty deodorant containers ready, standing upright with the lids removed on a piece of wax paper. Pour the deodorant mixture into the containers. This mixture will fill 2 deodorant containers with a bit left over, which you can pour into another container and apply with fingers or just save and add to the next batch.

This is a great recipe and won't leave greasy spots or stains on your clothing. You can add a different blend of essential oils if you prefer a different scent, but make sure to add the tea tree oil for its antiseptic properties.

Money-Saving Tip: If you do happen to get stains on your clothing, spot-treat right away with club soda. Follow up later when you are doing laundry with my homemade Stain Stick (page 112).

body scrubs

. . .

With all of these wonderful homemade beauty products, you'd think I'd be better at taking care of my skin, but being a wife and a mother, I rarely get more than a few minutes to myself.

When I realize how bad my skin has gotten, I know it's time to use a good scrub to refresh and invigorate my skin. But I'm not about to head to an expensive bath and beauty store to get these scrubs, because it is just way too easy and much more cost-effective to make them by using what I already have in my kitchen cupboards. One jar of my Lemon Poppy Seed Scrub costs about $2 to make. A similar scrub from a name-brand company costs over $20 per jar. That doesn't exactly fit in my budget!

I love all of these scrubs because they have a great cleansing power and a wonderful refreshing scent. They will invigorate your skin and your senses, perfect to get you ready for summer!

Lemon Poppy Seed Scrub

The sugar and the poppy seeds in this recipe will help scrub and exfoliate your skin.

——— WHAT YOU NEED ———

1 teaspoon poppy seeds
1 cup sugar
½ cup olive oil or coconut oil (extra-virgin if possible)
Juice and zest from 1 lemon
1 teaspoon honey

In a small bowl, mix together the poppy seeds and the sugar. If you are using coconut oil, warm it up first so it's easy to incorporate; olive oil can just be poured straight into the mixture. Add the oil, the juice and zest from the lemon, and the honey. Mix all the ingredients together until there are no clumps of any one ingredient.

To use, simply scrub anywhere on your body that you wish to remove dead or dry skin and invigorate. Rinse off after scrubbing.

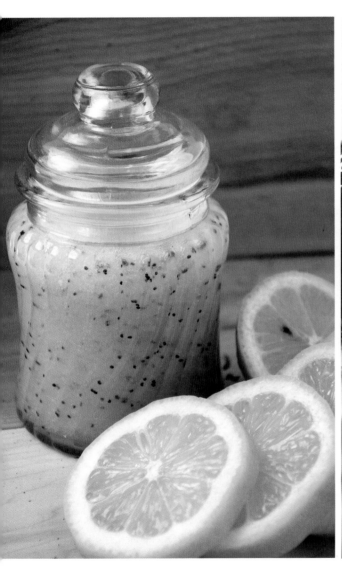
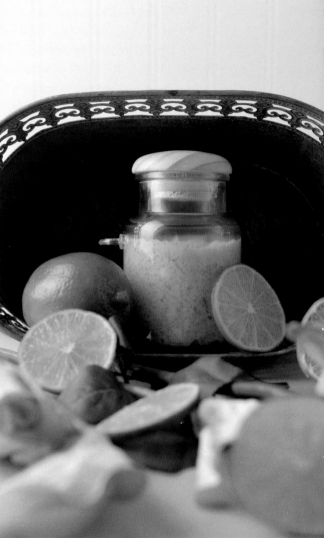

Coconut Lime Body Scrub

This is another great refreshing scrub. Its scent will leave you feeling invigorated and ready to go.

————————— WHAT YOU NEED —————————

1 cup sugar

½ cup coconut oil (extra-virgin if possible)

Juice and zest from 1 lime

1 teaspoon honey

In a small bowl, mix together all the ingredients until well blended. You may need to soften or melt the coconut oil before adding so it can be incorporated into the mixture. Place in a container and scrub onto skin as needed. Rinse off after using.

You can also substitute 2 tablespoons grapefruit juice for the lime in this recipe for a twist.

Make sure this recipe doesn't get too hot, as the coconut oil will separate from the sugar. Store in a cool dark place, ideally near the bathroom, until ready to use.

Oatmeal Cookie Body Scrub

This simple scrub is a fun one to give as a gift. It smells so good!

————————— WHAT YOU NEED —————————

½ cup uncooked old-fashioned oats

1 cup brown sugar

½ cup coconut oil (softened or melted, extra-virgin if possible)

Pulse the oats in a food processor for a few seconds until they are in very small pieces. Mix with the brown sugar and pour the coconut oil over the top. Mix all the ingredients together in a small bowl until incorporated. Place in a container and scrub onto skin as needed. Rinse off after using.

For a really decadent scrub, mix softened coconut butter into the recipe instead of coconut oil. It really makes it smell like cookies!

Money-Saving Tip: These scrubs make a great gift! You can pick up fun glass jars at the dollar store that are perfect to dress up your presentation.

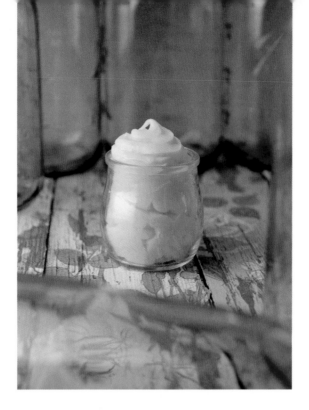

body butters

· · ·

For a good basic lotion, I stick to either my basic Whipped Coconut Oil Lotion (page 46) or Lotion Bars (page 63). But occasionally I like to have a fun, scented lotion for something special. I also love to give these body butters as gifts, either by themselves or in gift baskets. Each of these has a special scent and is incredibly moisturizing.

Since these body butters are easy to make, they are a fun project to do with friends. You can invite a couple of people over and have them each bring a few of the ingredients needed. Spend the afternoon creating unique body butters and then swap them so you all have a little of each kind.

Chocolate Body Butter

WHAT YOU NEED

1 cup coconut oil (extra-virgin if possible)
1 cup cocoa butter
¼ cup beeswax

In a saucepan on low heat, melt all the ingredients together. Pour into a medium bowl and place in the refrigerator until hardened (about 20 minutes). Whip with an electric hand mixer until soft and creamy. Place in a jar or container (this fits well in a wide-mouthed pint glass mason jar) and use as needed. If the mixture melts, simply re-whip when it hardens again. To prevent this from happening, store in a cool, dark place.

Shea Body Butter

WHAT YOU NEED

1 cup shea butter
½ cup coconut oil (extra-virgin if possible)
½ cup olive oil

In a saucepan on low heat, melt all the ingredients together until well blended. Pour into a medium bowl and place in the refrigerator until hardened (about 20 minutes). Remove the bowl from the fridge and whip the butter mixture with an electric hand mixer until soft and creamy. Place in a jar or container and use as needed.

Mango Body Butter

WHAT YOU NEED

1 cup shea butter
½ cup mango butter
½ cup olive or jojoba oil
5 drops cinnamon leaf essential oil
5 drops sweet orange essential oil

In a saucepan on low heat, melt the shea butter, mango butter, and olive or jojoba oil together, stirring until well blended. Remove from heat and add the essential oils. Pour into a medium bowl and place in the refrigerator until hardened (about 20 minutes). Whip the butter mixture with an electric hand mixer until soft and creamy. Place in a jar or container and use as needed.

Money-Saving Tip: It's fun to experiment with various butters (like mango butter, shea butter, and cocoa butter). If you buy some for another recipe and aren't sure what else to do with it, you can usually replace any other butter in a body recipe (e.g., replace shea butter with mango butter).

refreshing peppermint foot lotion

· · ·

Generally in the summer my feet remain one color: dirt brown. Washing doesn't seem to improve matters until the end of the gardening season. My feet work quite hard in the summer, from maneuvering around plants as I pick the fresh produce to standing in the kitchen for hours upon hours, preserving that same produce. The summer days are long for a reason here, because there is so much work to do before winter. The garden has to be cared for, the animals need extra attention since they are having babies, surplus produce needs to be preserved, and outbuildings and other parts of the little farmstead need to be kept up. I'm thankful for every extra minute of daylight.

After a long day on my feet, I try to sit down for a bit before heading to bed. Sometimes in the evenings I use some of my Refreshing Peppermint Foot Lotion to get them rested up for another long day.

This lotion is another one that is so simple to make, and you will love the results. The peppermint oil will leave your feet feeling revitalized after a long day. It also works great on sore muscles.

WHAT YOU NEED

1 tablespoon cocoa butter
¼ cup shea butter
2 tablespoons coconut oil (extra-virgin if possible)
1 tablespoon avocado oil
1 teaspoon vitamin E oil
¼ teaspoon peppermint essential oil

In a saucepan on low heat, melt together the cocoa butter, shea butter, and coconut oil. Remove from heat and mix in the avocado oil, vitamin E oil, and peppermint essential oil. Pour into a medium bowl and refrigerate until hardened (about 20 minutes). Whip the lotion with an electric hand mixer until light and creamy. Apply to feet as needed.

This is a great lotion following a detox foot bath, which couldn't be simpler to make.

Place ¼ cup Epsom salts, ¼ cup baking soda, and 1 teaspoon bentonite clay powder (optional) in a shallow container (big enough for your feet) and fill with several inches of warm water. Soak feet for about 20 minutes or until the water begins to cool. Make sure to drink plenty of water during this time. Follow your foot bath with the Refreshing Peppermint Foot Lotion.

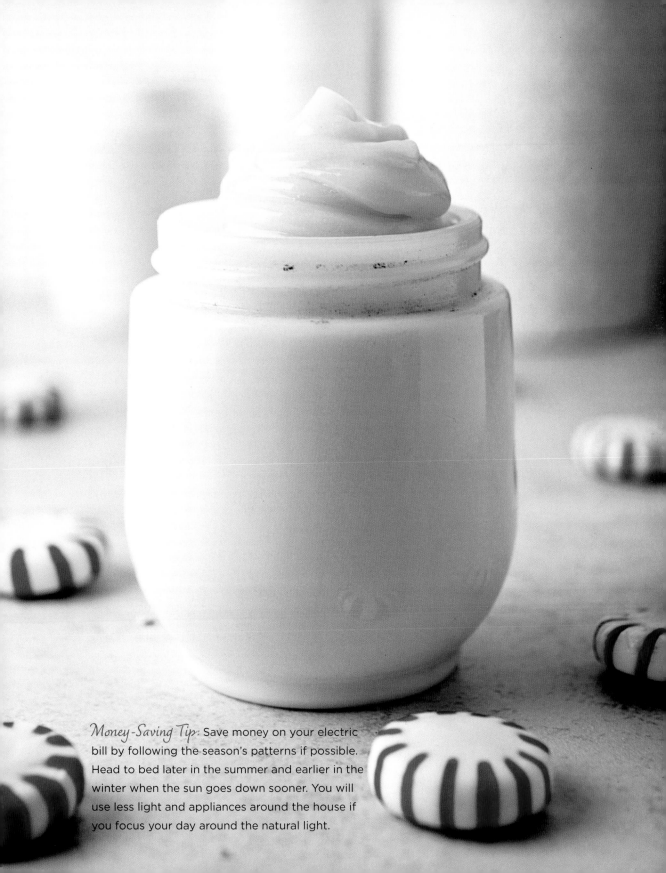

Money-Saving Tip: Save money on your electric bill by following the season's patterns if possible. Head to bed later in the summer and earlier in the winter when the sun goes down sooner. You will use less light and appliances around the house if you focus your day around the natural light.

cracked heel relief cream

. . .

I'm a barefoot kind of girl. In the summer you'll rarely find me with shoes on unless we have to make a trip to town, and I don't even own a pair of tennis shoes (we wear boots all winter). I love feeling the grass and the ground beneath my feet and being close to nature. Of course, this means that I tend to suffer from cracked heels fairly often. If you have similar issues, you know that it's not fun to have cracked, bleeding heels at any time of year.

Using the Cracked Heel Relief Cream is simple but requires patience. Your skin took its time getting that way and it's going to take a little time to heal. Thankfully, you should be able to see (and feel) results after just a few days. Pair this cream with a nice thick lotion (like the Lotion Bars, page 63, or the Eczema Cream, page 65) during the day and you should see even faster healing and healthier skin.

------ WHAT YOU NEED ------

½ cup raw honey

1 teaspoon avocado oil

1 tablespoon coconut oil (extra-virgin if possible)

Mix all the ingredients together in a small bowl. Rub on feet before bedtime and put socks on. Leave the mixture on all night and rinse off anything left in the morning. Follow the rinsing with a thick lotion and repeat nightly as needed until cracks begin to heal.

Money-Saving Tip: Raw honey is a little harder to find, but the added benefits over processed honey are worth it, especially if you plan to use it in lotions and healing creams. Look for raw or unprocessed honey at the grocery store or online or ask a local beekeeper if they have any that you might be able to purchase for less.

shoe and foot spray

· · ·

It's not a subject that one likes to talk about, but inevitably, someone in your family will have very smelly feet or unbelievably smelly shoes. You know that baking soda helps to remove smells, but who really wants baking soda–powdered feet?

We definitely have our fair share of smelly shoes. They aren't pleasant and give my tiny mudroom a very unpleasant odor, which I'd rather not share with company when they are walking through the door.

For these occasions, I developed this effective recipe. A few sprays in the shoes will help with the unpleasant odors. You can also spray it directly on feet to help kill the odor-causing bacteria. Either way, it really works!

———— **WHAT YOU NEED** ————

½ cup witch hazel

5 drops grapefruit essential oil

5 drops lemon essential oil

5 drops tea tree essential oil

5 drops lavender essential oil

Place all the ingredients in a small spray bottle. Shake to mix and spray as needed on feet and in shoes.

The lemon, tea tree, and lavender oils are all antifungal, to attack the source of the problem. Grapefruit oil adds an antibacterial punch to the mixture as well, helping to clear out any bad bacteria from the area where the spray is used. And of course, each of these oils has a great scent to help remove the odors from the area!

Money-Saving Tip: Shoes will last longer when they are free of bacteria and fungus. Using Shoe and Foot Spray at least once a week should help prolong the life of your shoes.

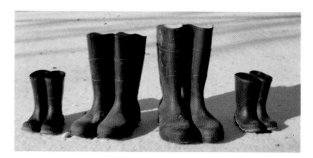

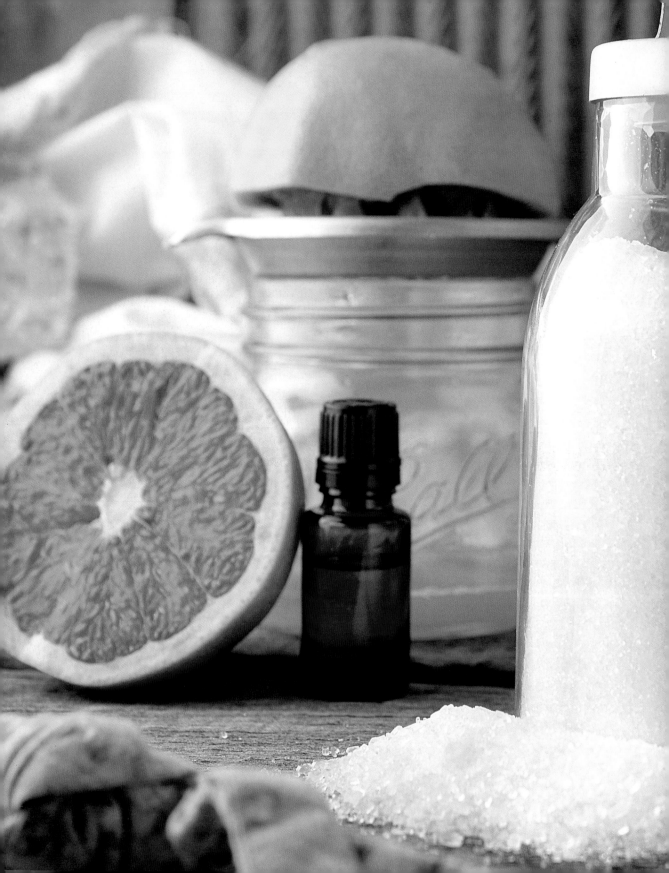

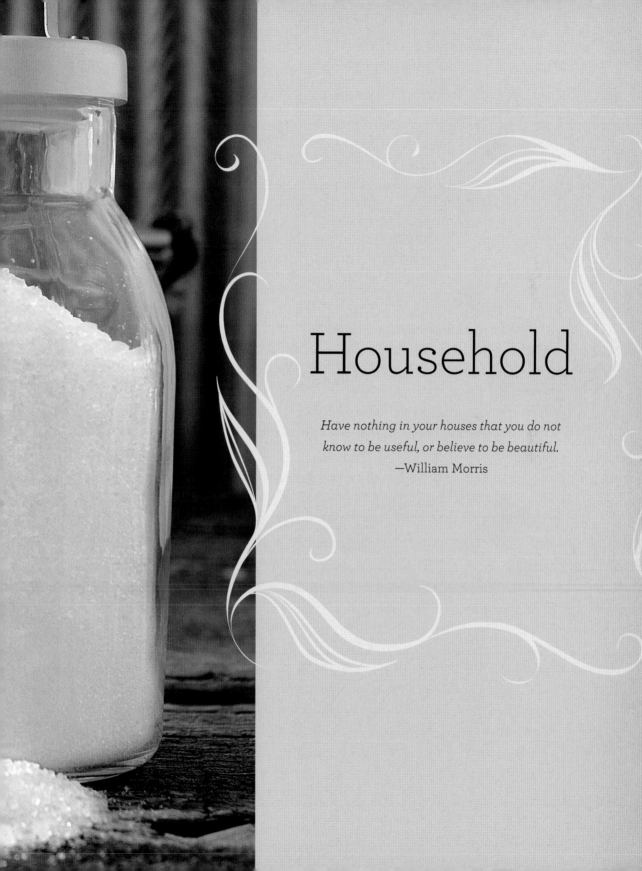

Household

*Have nothing in your houses that you do not
know to be useful, or believe to be beautiful.*
—William Morris

Believe it or not, I used to love cleaning my house. I would come home from work and spend my days off making sure that everything was spotless, the windows were washed, the clothes were always clean, and the dishwasher barely had any work to do.

Of course, that was in our pre-children days!

Now I'm lucky if I wash the windows a few times a year, laundry always seems like a weeklong affair, and just when I think I have it finished, I find a few pairs of dirty socks hidden behind the couch.

Life happens, and although I love my children to the end of the world, there is no denying the fact that they are messy little creatures. We've found several ways to keep the house mostly clean but there's not a day that goes by when it's perfect. But then . . . who really wants to strive for perfection anyway? Playing in the sandbox all afternoon with my little ones sounds like much more fun than chasing after them every second of the day to make sure that they aren't getting dirty. Not to mention that since we have livestock and a little farm . . . dirt and mess are inevitable.

I was spending a pretty penny on some natural, non-toxic cleaners when I realized just how easy it is to make everything myself at home. Plus I absolutely love having the ingredients on hand to make all kinds of cleaning products; it's not fun to have to go to the store for all-purpose cleaner to clean up after a sick little one when you yourself aren't feeling so great.

Household products can be one of the more frugal DIY items you make. They generally use the same basic ingredients and have very few ingredients, making them thrifty and something you can mix up in a snap.

Homemade cleaners and household products don't contain the powerful toxic chemicals that store-bought cleaners do, yet they are very effective. Take an item as simple as vinegar—an excellent disinfectant and deodorizer with grease-cutting power. Vinegar helps kill bacteria on hard surfaces such as *Salmonella* and *E. coli*. We've used vinegar as a base for many of our cleaners for years and have always been happy with the results. In this chapter you will find out how to make everything from your own produce wash spray to a recipe for dishwasher detergent.

Keeping a Simple Household

Something that's very important in our simple style of living is creating a household environment that's not stressful. No one wants to come home to a cluttered, disorganized house! Here are a few tips to get you started on creating a simple, nonstressful household no matter where you live.

KEEP THE CLUTTER TO A MINIMUM (aka: get rid of stuff!). After all of our big moves, we began seeing less and less of a need for the things that we'd acquired over our few years of marriage. They were hard to move around, hard to store, and just more work than they were worth. We started with one major cleanout, selling off about a quarter of everything we owned. I picked out things we never used or didn't need and sold them all. A few months later I did another big cleanout. This time we pulled out everything we still hadn't used since our last cleanout and sold all of that. We'd reduced our total household items by about 50 percent! Then we had one final cleanout. This time I kept only the things that we really needed and used on a daily or weekly basis and things that had very special meanings for us. Everything else was sold or donated.

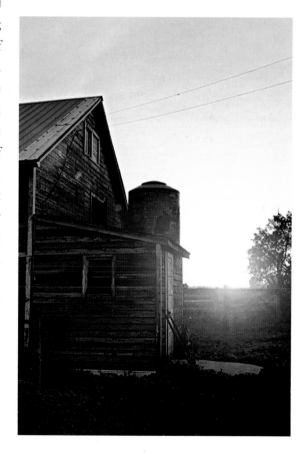

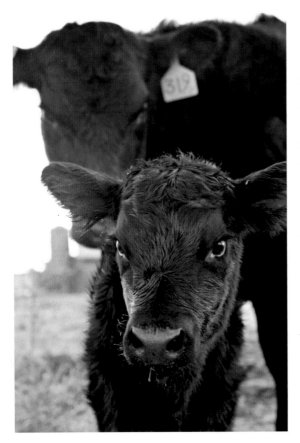

It's been a few years since we had this major cleanout and I can tell you one thing for sure . . . we don't miss a single item we got rid of. Plus now there isn't clutter in my home. We only have a few well-placed items for décor that either mean something to us or are useful. Drastically reducing our household items has been the single best thing that we've done on our path to simpler living.

CREATE SPACES FOR EVERYTHING. Since we live in a little house, I don't have any space to waste. Each room has many purposes and there is a space for everything. Sections of rooms often have a special purpose, like in our dining room we have a "go station" right by the door, with hats, bags, keys, and anything else we need when we are running out the door. If I can't find a place for something in our house, we don't keep it.

KEEP A CALM ENVIRONMENT. Not long after we moved into our little farmstead, I realized that mornings seemed hectic and created a stressful vibe for the rest of the day. I knew that if I could find a simple way to create peace in our home in the mornings, it would set the tone for the rest of the day. Now when I get up, I put on the coffee for my husband, I get breakfast ready and out on the table, I light a few well-placed candles in the dining room in my little lanterns, and I put on some soft, inspirational music. When the boys come downstairs for the day they are greeted by a peaceful environment. Since I try to plan our breakfasts ahead of time or the night before, it only takes me a few extra minutes to put this all together in the morning.

These are just a few tips you can try for creating a simpler, more peaceful household. Now let's get on to making some of these great household products so you can keep your home neat and tidy (or at least as neat and tidy as it can possibly be with a family!).

cooking spray

. . .

It's been years and years since I picked up a bottle of cooking spray from the grocery store. I think I remember buying it a long time ago, but it's just a distant memory. One that makes me wonder why I didn't think about my purchase first and realize how incredibly easy it would be to make my own spray. Cooking spray from the store usually costs over $4 per container and it doesn't seem to last very long. My homemade recipe costs around $0.50 per container (depending on the oil used) and usually lasts me several months.

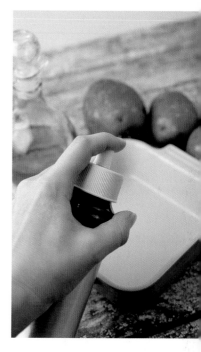

If you are able to find a special cooking spray bottle (kitchen stores and online retailers have them), all you will need to do is simply add your favorite oil (we use olive oil) and pump the bottle to create a pressurized spray. Nothing else needed!

If you prefer not to buy a special bottle and you happen to have an empty spray bottle sitting around at home that you can use, here's the simple recipe.

--- WHAT YOU NEED ---

1 cup filtered water

½ cup oil

Mix the water and oil together in your clean spray bottle. Spray the cooking spray onto your pans and bakeware using a fine mist spray setting. Make sure to shake the bottle before using. Store the bottle in a cool, dry place (such as a cupboard or kitchen pantry) until ready to use. You will want to use this mixture up within a month or two so the oil doesn't go rancid and give your foods an "off" taste.

When using any kind of cooking spray with baked goods, spray your pan with cooking spray first and then dust with a light coating of flour.

Money-Saving Tip: If you use a lot of oil in cooking and baking, make sure to buy large containers and skip the small, pricey bottles where you are paying for the packaging. We always try to buy oils in the gallon size.

dish soap

. . .

For the longest time, the thought of creating my own dish soap seemed intimidating. I wasn't quite sure on the amounts of ingredients I would need to get my dishes clean, and my previous attempts hadn't created good suds like a commercial dish soap.

But do suds = clean? Absolutely not! In fact, many of the suds and bubbles that we correlate with dish soap and "cleaning" are just a mixture of unnecessary chemicals. All we really need in a dish soap is cleaning power and degreasing power, and that's just what this homemade dish soap will create for you!

Fragrance-Free Dish Soap

——————— WHAT YOU NEED ———————

½ cup unscented castile soap   *1 tablespoon grated bar soap*
1 tablespoon baking soda   *1½ cups hot filtered water*

In a medium bowl, mix together the castile soap, baking soda, and grated bar soap. Slowly add the hot water over the soap mixture and stir until dissolved. Set the mixture on the counter to cool and stir as needed to make sure the ingredients are dissolved and mixed in. Place in an old hand soap or dish soap dispenser and use for washing dishes. For fragrance-free soap, make sure to use an unscented bar soap (we use an unscented castile bar soap).

Antibacterial Dish Soap

——————— WHAT YOU NEED ———————

½ cup unscented castile soap   *5 drops peppermint essential oil*
1 tablespoon baking soda   *5 drops ginger essential oil*
1 tablespoon grated bar soap   *1½ cups hot filtered water*

In a medium bowl, mix together the castile soap, baking soda, grated bar soap, and essential oils. Slowly pour the hot water over the soap mixture and stir until dissolved. Set the mixture on the counter to cool and stir as needed to make sure the ingredients are dissolved and mixed in. Grapefruit and ginger essential oils are antibacterial; however, if you prefer something different, you can also try tea tree, lavender, or rosemary essential oils.

Citrus Dish Soap

─────────────── WHAT YOU NEED ───────────────

½ cup citrus castile soap

1 tablespoon baking soda

1 tablespoon grated bar soap

10 drops sweet orange essential oil

1½ cups hot filtered water

In a medium bowl, mix together the castile soap, baking soda, grated bar soap, and sweet orange essential oil. Slowly add the hot water over the soap mixture and stir until dissolved. Set the mixture on the counter to cool and stir as needed to make sure the ingredients are dissolved and mixed in. Do not add any other citrus-scented essential oil to this soap, as most citrus oils can cause your skin to become phototoxic (extremely sensitive to sunlight). Sweet orange essential oil does not create photo-toxic reactions.

Doing the dishes is a great way to get your little ones involved in household projects and chores. When they are very young, you can teach them to do the dishes by letting them wash their play dishes in the sink, just like they would with real dishes. As time goes on and they get better at "playing dishes," you can start letting them help you wash the real dishes in the house. This homemade dish soap is great because it's gentle on even your little one's skin and you know it's safe for them to use.

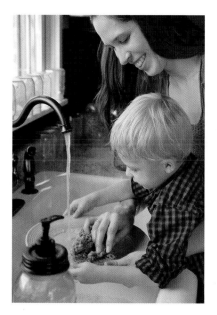

Money-Saving Tip: All out of dish soap and don't have the ingredients to make more? You can simply wash your dishes with vinegar. Mix a little vinegar with warm water in the sink, wash, and rinse. Any remaining vinegar scent will dissipate as the dishes dry.

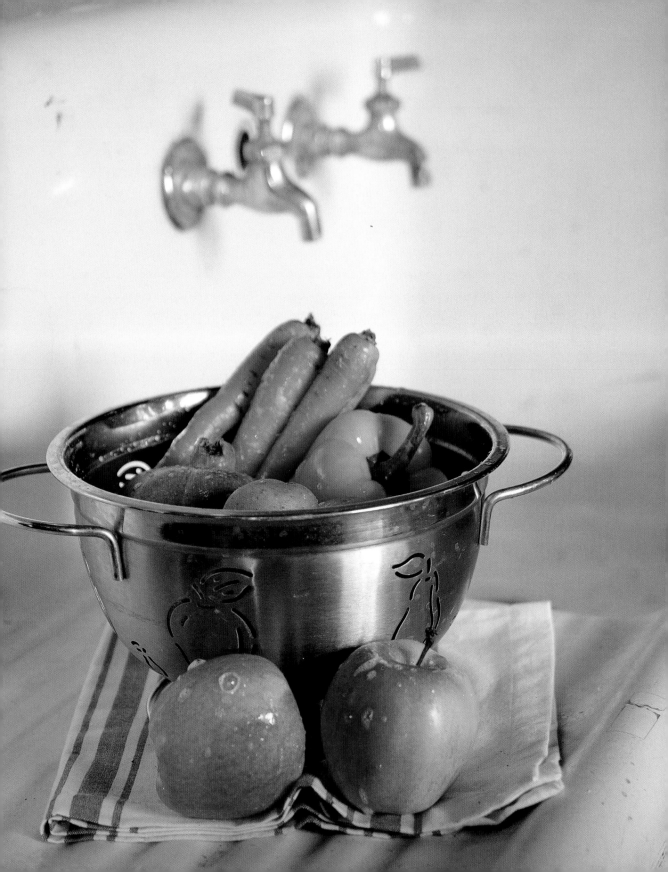

produce wash spray

. . .

This produce wash spray is yet another great helper in the kitchen that you can create easily. Thanks to everything from pesticides to bugs and dirt, it's best to wash your produce (whether from the store or from your garden). I know many people who don't wash their garden produce before eating, but for me, one taste of crunchy dirt and I would be done, so we wash first!

My little ones love to help wash produce when we bring it in from the garden. My older son will bring his stool over to the sink and be my "big helper" and help me scrub the produce clean. His favorite veggie to wash is potatoes because we let him use the potato scrub brush!

Adding a bit of grapefruit essential oil, which is naturally antibacterial, in this recipe gives it some great non-toxic cleaning power.

WHAT YOU NEED

1 tablespoon baking soda
¼ cup unscented castile soap
1 cup filtered water
5 drops grapefruit essential oil

In a medium bowl, mix together all the ingredients. Make sure that the baking soda has dissolved completely in the water before adding to a spray bottle. Add the mixture into a clean, empty spray bottle and spray on produce before washing.

To preserve your freshly purchased produce, you may also want to use a quick rinse after you bring them home. Simply add ½ cup of apple cider vinegar to a sinkful of cool water. Soak your produce (everything from apples to lettuce) in the vinegar rinse for a few minutes before removing and drying. This will help your produce last a bit longer until you are ready to use it, creating less food waste.

Money-Saving Tip: Save on produce by buying in season and shopping smart. Use farmers' markets for good deals on bulk produce, and in the winter, when seasonal produce is low and expensive, buy frozen vegetables. They are inexpensive and were flash frozen at the peak of their ripeness so they tend to have the most nutrients.

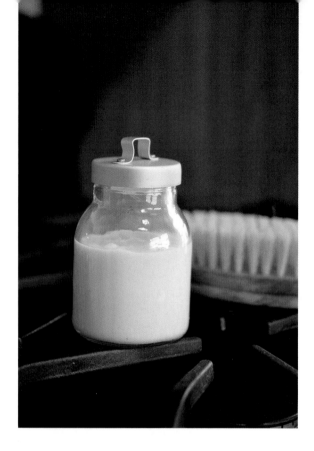

oven cleaner

· · ·

When we moved into the farmhouse, I bought a brand-new oven to put in our renovated kitchen. I'd never owned a gas oven before and we found a display model on clearance at our local appliance store. I loved that big beautiful thing and couldn't wait to use it after cooking in a tiny camper for the previous year. I was determined that I would never get it dirty and that I would always keep it shiny and clean . . . forever.

Well, of course you know that it doesn't really work that way. Butter drips out of pans, food falls onto the bottom of the oven while you are stirring a dish, and before you know it, the bottom of the oven is caked with some kind of black crusty scariness that may or may not have mostly been from your last attempt at butter cookies. It's not pretty and it doesn't smell good. Regular all-purpose chemical cleaners seem to have no effect, and I'm not sure about you, but I really would rather not spend all afternoon trying to scrub out my oven.

This homemade cleaner works like a charm! It has some serious scrubbing power and will get your oven looking shiny and new once again. This cleaning recipe also doubles as an excellent toilet bowl cleaner and will even remove hard water stains.

———————— WHAT YOU NEED ————————

¼ cup castile soap
¾ cup baking soda
10 drops tea tree essential oil
1 tablespoon ground pumice (optional)

In a bowl, mix together the castile soap, baking soda, and tea tree essential oil. You may need to add a bit more castile soap to get it to the right consistency. Store the mixture in an old bottle or container and use it to scrub any dirty surface such as your oven as needed. To use, simply spread the scrub mixture over the area that needs to be cleaned. Let it sit for a few minutes and then use a damp towel or sponge to scrub it off. If any scrub remains on the surface, wipe it off with a damp towel.

If you need a scrub that packs a powerful punch, add some ground pumice (which you can purchase online). You will need to add a bit of water to get the mixture to just the right consistency, but it will really give it great scrubbing power, perfect for the particularly stuck-on food in the oven. If you can't find pumice but still want scrubbing punch, add used coffee grounds.

Money-Saving Tip: Use your oven for many purposes. After you remove a dish from baking, warm items (on oven-safe dishes) for your next meal. You can even use your oven as an incubator for your homemade yogurt! To make homemade yogurt, heat ½ gallon of whole or 2 percent milk to 200 degrees on the stovetop (stirring constantly). Remove from heat and cool to 115 degrees (check the temps with a candy thermometer). Add in ½ cup of plain yogurt that contains live active cultures. Whisk together until smooth and pour into a half-gallon jar or oven-safe container. Place towels around the container or jar and set in the oven with the light on (do not turn the "Bake" setting on). Monitor your yogurt so that it stays at 110 degrees for at least 4 hours (longer for a thicker yogurt). When you are happy with the consistency, remove it from the oven and store in the refrigerator. If your family enjoys yogurt often like ours does, this could be a huge cost savings!

dishwasher detergent

· · ·

Quite frankly, I was excited about not having a dishwasher in our farmhouse. (There was just not enough room in my very tiny kitchen!) I'd never really had luck with using one because we'd only lived in places that had hard water, and if you have hard water, you know that it just ruins a dishwasher in a short amount of time. In our previous home, every dishwasher would work only a year or so before it gave up, and no amount of cleaning and scrubbing kept the hard water deposits away.

So when my dishwasher-owning friends began asking me for a dishwasher detergent recipe that worked, I turned to someone who had a dishwasher that worked and who I knew created just as many recipes from scratch as I did—my mom. This is her recipe to keep your dishes sparkling.

WHAT YOU NEED

1 cup washing soda
¼ cup citric acid
⅛ cup sea salt
5 drops lemon essential oil
5 drops grapefruit essential oil

In a bowl, mix all the ingredients together until blended. Store in a jar or container until ready to use. Use as you would commercial dishwasher detergent in your dishwasher and place a small amount of vinegar in the "rinse" cup.

For hard water you may need to adjust the recipe a bit, adding a little more citric acid and lemon essential oil. This recipe may not work for extremely hard water.

Money-Saving Tip: Make sure to keep your dishwasher clean to keep it running at tip-top shape so that it will last as long as possible and not need as many repairs. We went through three dishwashers within three years at our old house because we didn't know how to keep them clean! Every month or so, place a glass cup full of vinegar upright on one of the shelves and run a cycle with the rest of the dishwasher empty to get it clean.

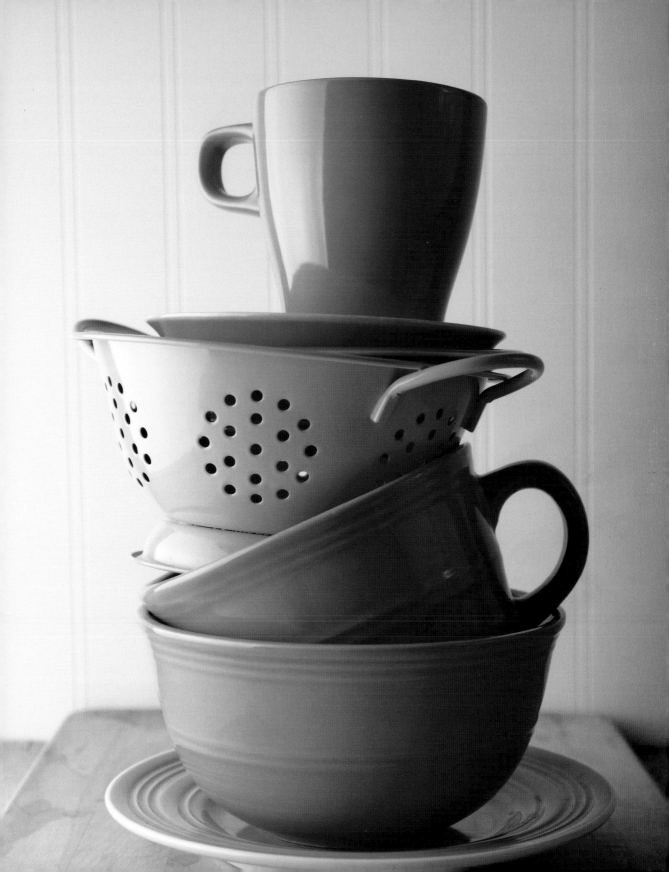

dusting spray

· · ·

It's one of my pet peeves to be dusting my house and to wipe the same area over and over, only to see half the dust flying around in the air and the other half still sitting on the counter that I was trying to wipe. To my mind, it just seems counterproductive and certainly doesn't help me get the job done any faster or enjoy it any more.

I remember when I was growing up that sometimes on cleaning day we would use some chemical-filled aerosol can of dusting spray to clean up our surfaces in the house and while that helped actually pick up the dust, there is no way I would want the added chemicals in the air in my house today.

But . . . can you believe it? You can make your own dusting spray from scratch, of course! This recipe is so easy that you will never grab another bottle of dusting spray at the store again; in fact, after reading this section you won't even have a need to enter the cleaning products aisle at the store ever again. Isn't it amazing how with just a few basic household items we can make everything we need? So let's make some dusting spray today.

─────────── WHAT YOU NEED ───────────

¼ cup vinegar (white or apple cider)
¾ cup oil (we use olive oil)
15 drops lemon essential oil

───────────────────────────────

Pour the vinegar, oil, and lemon essential oil into a clean, empty spray bottle. Shake to combine ingredients before using and spray on surfaces that are dusty. Wipe up with a dry towel or cloth. This spray also will act as a simple furniture polish, but for an even more protective finish, you also might want to use the Furniture Polish (page 98). Vinegar is a great disinfectant as well, so you will also be killing germs as you are cleaning.

My kids absolutely love to help with the dusting! I just spray a bit of the home-made dusting spray on their towels and they love to wipe down anything in sight. (Of course, we direct them toward the things that actually need to be dusted, but it's all part of the learning process!) We have a couple "methods to our madness" when it comes to dusting. We usually just dust one room per day so it doesn't get tiring, and the whole family helps, so it takes about two minutes to do. Plus we have hardly any knickknacks or clutter around our home, which are the things that generally take the most time to dust around.

Money-Saving Tip: If you aren't buying vinegar in bulk, it's time to start now! Vinegar can be used in so many different household applications, from cleaning the bathroom to baking! As with oil, if you buy the small bottles, you are paying for packaging, so go for the gallon jugs.

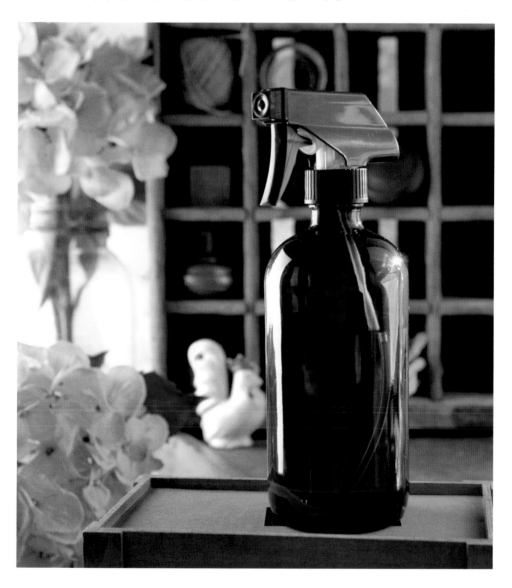

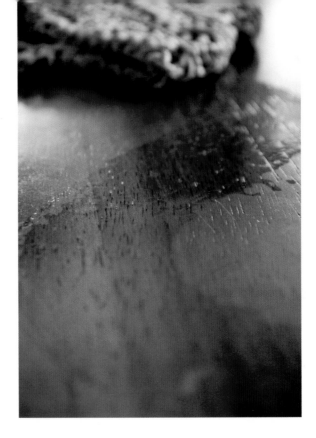

furniture polish

. . .

Has your furniture started to look a bit the worse for wear? In our seven years of marriage, my husband and I haven't been able to afford many new pieces of furniture, so we look for used furniture in good condition that we can spruce up on our own. It's pretty amazing what a good furniture polish can do, even for a piece that looks like it's beyond repair.

When we moved into the farmhouse, due to our circumstances (previously living in a camper), we had no furniture. A few weeks after we moved in, I found a used farm-style table made of solid, good-quality wood selling for just $60 that we instantly fell in love with. The table was in rough shape from decades of wear, but I whipped up some of my furniture polish and cleaned it from top to bottom. The first time I sent a picture of our new dining room to family, everyone went absolutely wild over our "amazingly beautiful new table"!

This polish recipe is very quick to make and will work wonders on your furniture (it works best on wood). Just grab the few items below from your kitchen and polish away.

────────────── WHAT YOU NEED ──────────────

2 black tea bags
1 cup warm filtered water
1 teaspoon beeswax, melted
1 teaspoon olive oil
¼ cup white or apple cider vinegar
5 drops lemon essential oil

Start by steeping the tea bags in the warm water for about 5 minutes. Cool slightly until the tea is cool enough to handle and wipe down any furniture that is to be polished with the strong tea mixture first. This will help remove any old polish from your furniture before you get started.

In a small bowl, mix together the melted beeswax, oil, vinegar, and lemon essential oil. Test on a small, inconspicuous part of your furniture first. If you're satisfied that it won't harm the finish, place a small amount on a soft towel and wipe onto your furniture. Do not wipe off. If there are any spots of excess oil, wipe them off with a dry, soft towel.

Money-Saving Tip: Be sure to polish your furniture a few times a year to keep it in the best shape possible so it will last. Buying new furniture is expensive, and it's simple to keep old furniture in great shape with a little love and homemade natural furniture polish!

floor cleaner

· · ·

When we arrived at our farmhouse after signing the papers, the first thing I did was run upstairs and rip up the carpet in the bedroom. I'd been crossing my fingers, hoping that underneath the dingy carpeting, the original 125-year-old hardwood floors would still be intact and that we'd be able to refinish them. I remember running back down the steep stairs and announcing proudly to my husband, "They are there and they are beautiful!"

After a ridiculous amount of sanding and resanding, the floors were resurfaced and back to their 1890 glory. They aren't perfect and they show their age in many spots, but I think they are lovely and really fit in with the feel of our house. We were able to refinish the floors in all the rooms but the kitchen, and although my husband will tell you for days how difficult it was to restore them, I know that he loves having them in here just as much as I do.

The floor cleaner recipe below will work on floors that are able to be cleaned with a cleaning agent or with water, but be sure to test it on a small area of your floors before using.

─────────── WHAT YOU NEED ───────────

1 cup filtered water
¼ cup vinegar (white or apple cider)
2 tablespoons rubbing alcohol
10 drops grapefruit essential oil
5 drops lemon essential oil

Combine all the ingredients in a spray bottle. Spray onto floors and hard surfaces to clean and disinfect. Wipe off with a dry towel. The vinegar cleans the floor (the smell will dissipate shortly), the alcohol keeps the spray from leaving any water marks on the floor, and the essential oils help disinfect germs and leave your floors smelling fresh and clean!

Money-Saving Tip: There's no need to buy expensive mops and floor-cleaning kits. A plain, cheap broom will do most of what you need, and mopping the floor with a few rags won't cost you anything.

cleaning wipes

· · ·

Busy moms sometimes don't have time to pull out a full brigade of cleaning products to get the house clean, especially when a family member is sick or when you are simply trying to do a quick tidy-up before company comes over.

I love having these cleaning wipes ready to use when a family member is sick; they're ideal for wiping off doorknobs, handles, and other places that germs can accumulate. I don't have to dig through all my cleaners and I still get the job done quickly (and can simply toss away the toweling afterward). Here are two versions of handy cleaning wipes. The first recipe is perfect for cleaning up after a sick household and the second is perfect for cleaning in a hurry before company comes over. Both are great to have on hand!

Make sure to use a thicker paper towel for this recipe so your wipes do not fall apart when you are trying to use them.

Antibacterial Cleaning Wipes

——————— WHAT YOU NEED ———————

1 roll paper towels
¼ cup vinegar
¼ cup filtered water
5 drops clove or tea tree essential oil
5 drops cinnamon bark essential oil
5 drops eucalyptus essential oil

Remove the cardboard tube from the center of the paper towel roll. Using a bread knife, cut the roll of paper towels in half so that you have two short rolls. Pull up a small corner of paper towel from the middle of the roll to get the wipes started. Place each half roll of towels in a container or a bag (old baby wipe containers work really well). In a small bowl, mix together the water, vinegar, and essential oils. Place half of the liquid mixture in the bottom of each container or bag. (This recipe will make enough for both halves of the paper towel roll.)

Let the toweling sit in the mixture until it soaks it up, then your cleaning wipes are ready to use!

Citrus Cleaning Wipes

If you'd rather have a citrus-based cleaning wipe, simply replace the essential oils in the recipe on page 101 (clove, cinnamon bark, and eucalyptus) with 10 drops of sweet orange essential oil and 5 drops lemon essential oil. You could also use lime, grapefruit, or bergamot essential oils in the same quantities for an alternative citrus-based cleaner.

Money-Saving Tip: Convenience sometimes isn't worth it. If you don't plan on using these wipes often, stick with the less-expensive homemade All-Purpose Cleaner (page 103).

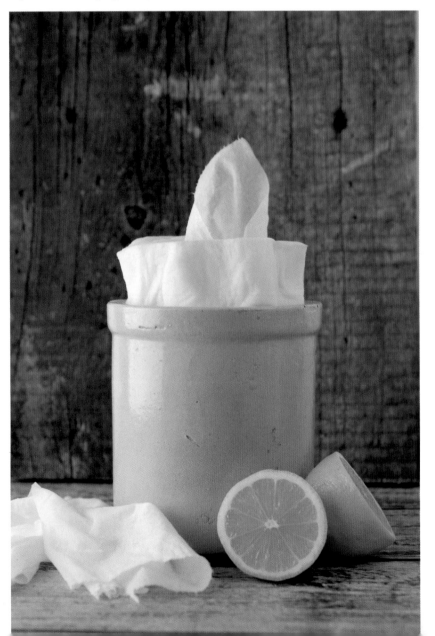

all-purpose and window cleaner

Every household needs to have a good all-purpose cleaner. At our house it tends to get daily use, cleaning up everything from dirt tracked in the dining room to tomato splatters on the kitchen cabinets. It's great for so many different things . . . I've even used it to clean up spots in my carpet when I didn't have any carpet cleaner mixed up!

As with most cleaners, you should test on a small area of what you plan on cleaning before you wipe down a large section. This cleaner will work great on most hard and soft surfaces but could possibly remove things like paint. Usually I find that on any surface where I cannot use the cleaner, such as a painted windowsill, a simple towel with water will get the job done instead.

The addition of tea tree or lavender essential oil in this recipe means the spray has antibacterial qualities, making it perfect for cleaning the bathroom or other germ-filled areas of the home.

All-Purpose Cleaner

WHAT YOU NEED

½ cup vinegar (white or apple cider)
1 cup filtered water
5 drops tea tree or lavender essential oil
10 drops sweet orange or grapefruit essential oil

Mix together all the ingredients in a clean, empty spray bottle. Spray directly on the surface of what you are trying to clean and wipe off with a dry towel.

Add a few drops of lemon essential oil to this cleaner to help remove sticky things.

For a window or glass cleaner, you won't need the essential oils so the recipe is basically the same, but make sure to use white vinegar. We've used the glass cleaner to clean up everything from our mirrors in the house to our dirty barn windows. It works perfectly!

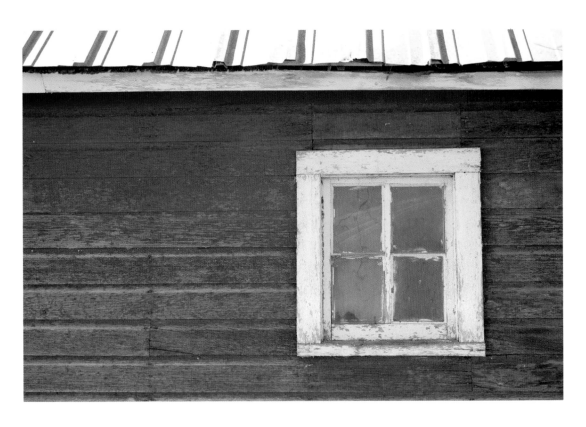

Window Cleaner

———————— WHAT YOU NEED ————————

½ cup white vinegar

1 cup filtered water

Mix ingredients together in a clean, empty spray bottle. Shake before using. Spray directly on glass and wipe off with a dry microfiber towel.

Money-Saving Tip: These cleaners can be used for more than just windows and surfaces in a pinch. I've used them for cleaning rugs, walls, and just about everything else when I didn't feel like mixing up another cleaning recipe!

carpet cleaner and shampoo

· · ·

Even though the floors in our farmhouse are mostly wood, I do have a few large rugs in a couple of the rooms to save our feet from getting too cold in the winter. With little ones who think it's quite fun to squish peach fruit snacks into the floor, having a good carpet cleaner is still a must.

This great recipe will work on most carpets, but as with all cleaners, you will definitely want to do a spot check first to make sure it's not going to discolor your carpet. If you do have issues with discoloration, leave the peroxide out of the mixture and see if that makes a difference. Also make sure to use a clear or uncolored dish soap in this recipe.

This recipe will work as a spot cleaner or as carpet shampoo in a shampooing machine.

───────── WHAT YOU NEED ─────────

¼ cup vinegar
1 tablespoon Dish Soap (page 88)
1 tablespoon hydrogen peroxide (optional)
Warm filtered water

Pour the vinegar, dish soap, and hydrogen peroxide into your carpet shampooer, fill the rest of the shampoo cavity with warm water, and use the shampooer as normal.

To use this recipe as a spot cleaner, simply mix the vinegar, dish soap, and hydrogen peroxide with 1 cup warm water. Use on smaller spots of carpet as needed.

For another supersimple spot treatment, sprinkle the spot on the carpet with baking soda, spray with vinegar, and let the chemical reaction take place. Then scrub the spot with an old brush and wipe up any excess soda with a wet towel.

Money-Saving Tip: Use an old toothbrush to spot-clean your carpet with this cleaning recipe.

laundry detergent

. . .

Clothes get DIRTY at our house. Between the mud puddles, taking care of animals and chores, and working in the garden, I don't think a day goes by without at least one outfit change necessitated by mud and dirt. I don't mind at all; a little dirt won't hurt anyone and it's all part of the country living experience! I do, however, prefer not to have to continually buy new clothes because of something getting ruined.

Have you ever thought of how blessed you are by having a washing machine or the ability to access a washing machine? In the Little House on the Prairie books, we read, of course, about how they washed laundry by hand with a harsh lye soap that made their eyes and hands sting. I'm so thankful that we don't have to do things like this anymore and can simplify our lives by using a modern washing machine!

We keep a minimal amount of clothing in our home mostly because we don't have closets so we don't have the storage space. But with the clothing I do keep, I usually have play/chore clothes for each person. These are a few outfits that are okay to get dirty and are not for wearing to town or church.

With all our clothes, but especially with the play clothes, we need a good laundry detergent that is easy to make. I've seen many versions of homemade detergent over the years, but this is what works for us and what gets our clothes clean.

This recipe makes a large batch, so if you are just trying it out to see if it will work for you, you may want to cut it in half. I prefer to make a large amount at one time because it keeps well and saves me time!

―――――――――― WHAT YOU NEED ――――――――――

2 bars castile soap

1¼ cups baking soda

1 cup citric acid

3 cups washing soda

½ cup sea salt

Start by grating the castile soap. Place the grated soap in a bowl and add the rest of the ingredients. Mix well so that all the ingredients are blended and you don't have any large clumps of a single ingredient. Use 1 tablespoon of laundry detergent per load of clothing. You may need to use a bit more if clothing is very dirty or if you have a top-loading washer.

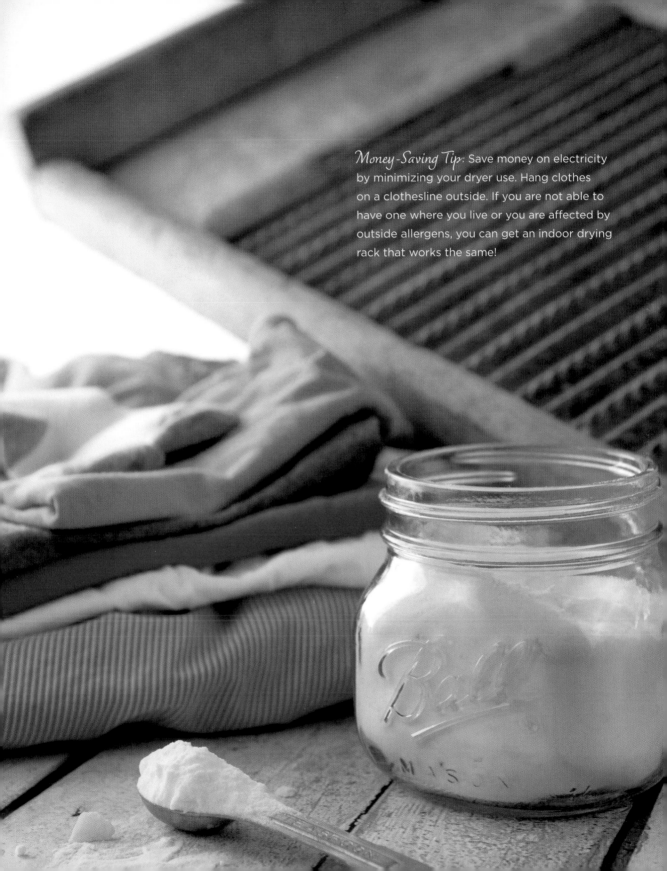

Money-Saving Tip: Save money on electricity by minimizing your dryer use. Hang clothes on a clothesline outside. If you are not able to have one where you live or you are affected by outside allergens, you can get an indoor drying rack that works the same!

fabric softener

. . .

With my homemade laundry detergent I usually find that I don't need a fabric softener, but it's nice to use occasionally, especially when washing jeans or other stiff clothing, or if you plan on line-drying your clothes. Fabric softener doesn't need to have scent but it can, and best of all, you can create it in the scent of your personal choice.

Fabric softener's main job is to soften the fabric of the garments and it's actually a very simple thing to do. All you need is a bit of salt! Epsom salt usually costs around $1 per pound. One pound of salt will soften many loads of laundry and last quite a while. You may be able to find coarse sea salt for even less and that will work the same as Epsom salts. That's what's great about this recipe, you can use what you have on hand at the time or whatever kind of salt is cheaper!

WHAT YOU NEED

Epsom salts or coarse sea salt

To soften fabric, simply add about 2 tablespoons of Epsom salt or coarse sea salt to each load of laundry. If you use my homemade Laundry Detergent (page 106), you may not need fabric softener at all, because the detergent already has salt in it.

Now, if you want to add a little scent in your load of laundry, nothing could be easier. You just need to create a special scent and add the essential oils to the salt. Here's one of our favorite blends:

Scented Fabric Softener

WHAT YOU NEED

1 cup salt (Epsom salts or sea salt)
5 drops grapefruit essential oil
5 drops ginger essential oil

Mix the salt and the oils together in a small bowl. Add 3 tablespoons of the mixture to each load of laundry. You can add the same amount of essential oil in any combination that is your favorite.

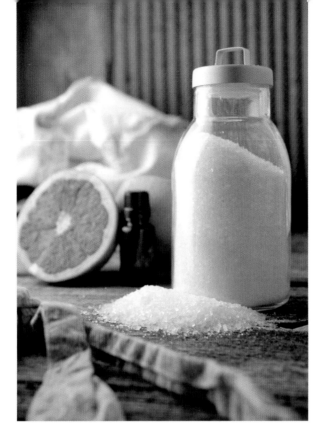

One more fabric softener recipe . . . if you need a softener with a bit of brightening power, you may enjoy the mixture below. You can add any of your favorite essential oils for scent.

Brightening Fabric Softener

WHAT YOU NEED

1 cup Epsom salts or sea salt
¼ cup baking soda
10 drops of your favorite essential oils

Mix together and add 3 tablespoons of the mixture to each load of laundry as needed.

Money-Saving Tip: You shouldn't need to use fabric softener with every load of laundry; just add it to the loads of jeans or other garments that have a tendency to get stiff after washing, especially if you plan to hang the clothes to dry.

wrinkle release and
fabric freshener spray

· · ·

Let me tell you something that you may not know. When you keep clothing in a camper or apartment or any small space for any period of time, you will have wrinkly clothes *all the time*. When we lived in the camper, I don't think a day went by when I didn't feel like a wrinkly mess. And washing didn't help. We had a tiny washer-dryer combo inside our camper, which was a very nice convenience and got our clothing clean, but it didn't help with the wrinkles unless I dried one single piece at a time. Not to mention it took about three hours to wash one tiny load of clothing. That's something I really don't miss!

No matter where you live and how you wash your clothing, wrinkles happen, especially in clothing that has been sitting in a drawer for a while. This Wrinkle Release Spray will help solve all your wrinkly needs!

Wrinkle Release Spray

—————— WHAT YOU NEED ——————

¼ cup homemade Fabric Softener (page 108)
1½ cups hot filtered water

In a bowl, mix the fabric softener and hot water. Stir the mixture until the softener dissolves completely. Pour the mixture into a clean, empty spray bottle. When needed, shake the bottle to mix and spray on wrinkled clothing while slightly stretching the garment.

If your garments are starting to smell like something that came out of the back of your grandma's closet, you may want to add a bit of scent to your Wrinkle Release and *voilà*! You have Fabric Freshener Spray!

Fabric Freshener Spray

WHAT YOU NEED

¼ cup homemade Fabric Softener (page 108)
1½ cups hot filtered water
8 drops essential oils

In a bowl, mix the fabric softener and hot water. Stir until the softener dissolves completely. If you've used scented fabric softener, you won't need to add more essential oils, but if you only have unscented fabric softener on hand, add your favorite essential oils now. Pour the mixture into a clean, empty spray bottle. When needed, shake the bottle to mix and spray on wrinkled clothing while slightly stretching the garment.

Make sure to use a clear (not dark-colored) essential oil for this recipe or you may get spots on your clothing.

Money-Saving Tip: Wearing your clothes often will ensure that clothing doesn't hang in the back of your closet and gather a "Granny's closet" smell. To accomplish this, work on keeping a minimalist closet and only keep the clothing that you need and wear often. Pack away seasonal clothing in boxes and totes until it needs to be worn. You could also make some simple lavender or herb sachets to tuck into the boxes to help keep your clothing smelling fresh and to help repel mice.

stain stick

. . .

No doubt about it, our lifestyle is hard on clothing. No matter how careful I am, I always seem to get something on my clothing, especially oil, even if I'm wearing an apron. In fact, I think I have a knack for getting some kind of oil on every new outfit I buy, which could be why I rarely buy new clothing and prefer to stick to used clothing instead.

This is one of my very favorite household recipes, and I think you'll love these handy little stain sticks as much as I do. They are easy to make, last a long time (so you won't have to make them often), and work like a charm. They really do get the stains out of clothing, even coconut oil!

Note: Washing soda is similar to baking soda but with a slightly different chemical makeup. You can find it near the laundry detergents at most stores. If you really can't find it at all, you can replace it with baking soda in this recipe; however, the recipe will "puff up" slightly, so just be aware when you are creating your recipe and make sure to use at least a medium-size saucepan if you are making this with the baking soda replacement.

WHAT YOU NEED
---

1 bar castile soap, grated

½ cup washing soda

2 tablespoons vinegar

4 tablespoons filtered water

2 tablespoons Dish Soap (page 88)

10 drops lemon essential oil

Melt the castile soap in a saucepan on medium-low heat. Mix in the washing soda, vinegar, and water, and stir until combined. Remove from heat and add the dish soap and essential oil. Pour or spoon the mixture into an empty, clean deodorant container. Spot-treat stains as needed before washing. Simply rub a bit of stain stick on the spot and let it sit anywhere from a few minutes to a few hours before washing the garment. This recipe will make enough for one stain stick.

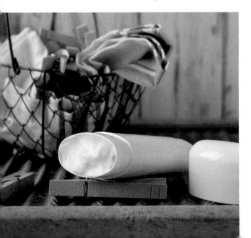

Money-Saving Tip: Wearing an apron isn't old-fashioned—it can help save your clothes! Why spend more on clothing than you need to? To keep your clothes from getting really stained up, make sure you have an apron or two on hand for baking, crafting, gardening, and other messy chores. Little ones can wear aprons too!

ant spray

· · ·

When we renovated our 125-year-old farmhouse, we found all kinds of things in the walls . . . postcards, old pictures, even a complete beehive that went from the main floor up into the second story! What we didn't find right away were the ants.

When spring hit I started noticing a few tiny ants on the kitchen floor. Just one here and there, nothing too alarming—or so it seemed. Our toddler thought it was funny to watch the bugs crawl around and I didn't put much thought into it since it was only the occasional, tiny ant. How bad could it get?

Then one day I woke up and went into the kitchen to find ants covering the floor and crawling up the cabinets! Either they had multiplied in a big way or the rest of their ant friends had suddenly decided to have a party on my kitchen floor. Since this incident, we have tried several different homemade methods to get them out and we've added more caulk to our baseboards to try to seal them out of the kitchen for good. Nothing worked, until we developed this spray.

While reading about the different methods of ant removal, I learned that ants hate cucumbers. Cucumbers are toxic to the food that ants normally like to feed on, so ants avoid cucumbers like the plague. In the summer we always have cucumbers when the garden is producing, so this seemed like a great and healthy method to keep the ants away! Of course, being the frugal family that we are, and because we happen to enjoy cucumbers very much, we prefer to use just the peels in our ant spray.

Peppermint is another ingredient that ants avoid because they hate the strong scent. Add vinegar (the last in the trifecta of things they can't stand!) and you've got a powerhouse spray that will keep your kitchen pest-free.

——————— WHAT YOU NEED ———————

Peels from 1 cucumber
1 cup warm filtered water
15 drops peppermint essential oil
¼ cup vinegar

Scatter the cucumber peels on a baking sheet and bake them in the oven at 400 degrees for about 5 to 10 minutes (but don't burn them!), until they are completely

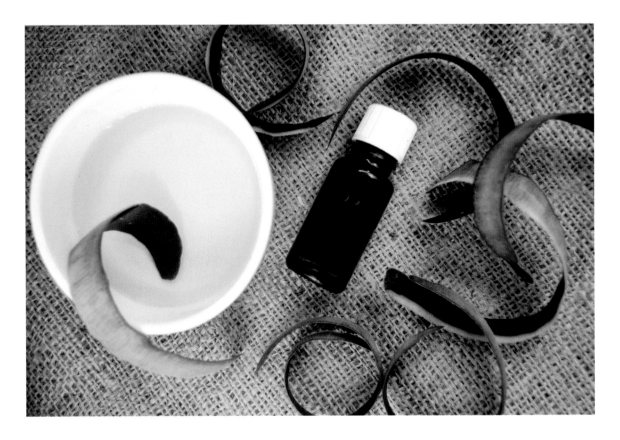

dried like a potato chip. Remove them from the oven and let them cool for a minute. In a food processor or blender, process the dried peels until you have a powder.

Pour the water, the peppermint essential oil, and the vinegar into an empty spray bottle. Using a funnel, pour in the cucumber peel powder. Shake the mixture thoroughly to dissolve the powder in the water.

Use this spray anywhere you have seen ants or don't want to see ants in the future! Spray along baseboards and floors to provide a line of defense for your kitchen and any other areas through which they might be entering your home. Repeat as needed to keep them from coming back.

Money-Saving Tip: Pesticides and insecticides (bug poisons) are expensive and dangerous to have in your home, around your family, or around pets. Experiment first with vinegar and various essential oils to eliminate the problem before you turn to store-bought chemicals. Most bug problems can be fixed naturally and by using things you already have on hand!

garden pest spray

· · ·

Gardening is a way of life for our family. If we didn't have a nice large garden in the summer, we wouldn't have very much fresh produce in the winter, or would have to spend a lot of money to get it. In addition to having a garden for ourselves, we also hope to maintain a small CSA (community supported agriculture) weekly produce basket from our little farm in the near future.

We grow all our produce without using any chemicals. Of course, when I have worked so hard to create a garden and it's so important to the family and essential in our lifestyle, I'll do anything to keep the bugs away—that is, I'll do anything but spray chemicals on my plants. I've tried a few different insecticidal soaps and sprays over the years but none worked as well as this essential oil blend. We've used this on all types of plants and bugs in our garden.

My recipe is rather concentrated, so it's a powerful bug spray. Depending on the pests you are fighting, you might find that you can either add a little bit more water to stretch it further, or you might use a little less water if you need a superpowerful formula.

Note: This spray will repel squash bugs in their "youth" stage but won't offer protection against them when they are fully grown. So make sure to spray at the first sight of squash bugs, and spray often.

All-Purpose Pest Spray

———————— WHAT YOU NEED ————————

1 cup filtered water
¼ cup oil (I use grapeseed)
20 drops rosemary essential oil
20 drops peppermint essential oil
20 drops clove essential oil
20 drops thyme essential oil

Pour all the ingredients into a spray bottle. Shake thoroughly to mix, and shake the bottle each time before spraying on plants. To apply, spray on leaves of the plants or directly at bugs in the morning or at least 12 to 24 hours before watering.

Quick Pest Spray

Here's a superquick spray that doesn't use any oils but will chase the pests away for a short time. Simply fill an 8-ounce spray bottle with filtered water and add ½ teaspoon of garlic powder. Shake well and spray on bugs when the powder has dissolved into the water. Do not spray on plants in the heat of the day; use in the morning or evening. This solution works in a pinch, but for a longer-lasting solution we prefer the essential oil blend above.

Aphid Spray

If you have an aphid problem, this simple spray will remove them from trees and plants. In the blender, put 1 cup diced fresh onion and 1 cup filtered water. Blend to a watery puree. You may need to add a little more water to make it sprayable, or you can simply sprinkle it over plants that are affected by aphids. Do not use on plants in the heat of the day; apply in the morning or evening.

Money-Saving Tip: A good dish soap can work wonders as a garden spray. For a bug, mold, or pest problem you aren't sure how to solve, start by mixing about ¼ cup of Dish Soap (page 88) with 16 ounces of filtered water and spraying on plants in the evening after watering. You might just find that's all you need!

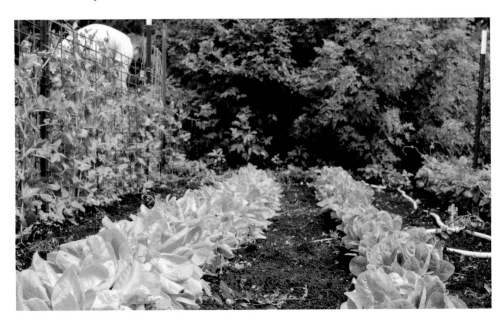

weed spray

· · ·

Not only do we have the joy of dealing with garden pests in the summer but we also have all sorts of lovely weeds. During our first summer in the farmhouse, I discovered all the little places, outside and inside, that the weeds will grow, including our mudroom. If weeds are large or not very plentiful, I usually just pull them up by hand, but for weeds that are growing in hard-to-reach places like sidewalks or driveways, it's easier to use a weed spray.

Keep in mind that this spray will kill not only weeds but grass, or anything else growing nearby, so watch where you spray it. The spray will work best if sprayed in the heat of the day, when the sun can also lend its weed-killing power.

WHAT YOU NEED

1 cup warm filtered water

¼ cup salt

1 tablespoon baking soda

2 cups vinegar

In a bowl, mix the warm water, salt, and baking soda. Stir until the soda and salt are completely dissolved. Add the vinegar and pour into a spray bottle. Spray directly at weeds as needed. Reapply a few times per day until the weeds have died.

Money-Saving Tip: Not all weeds are bad. Take a class or gather some information about your local plants for foraging. You will be amazed what's growing in your yard that is delicious and can be beneficial to your diet!

gel air fresheners

. . .

Wouldn't it be nice to have a pleasant scent in your home without the use of candles or heavily fragranced chemical products from the store? We like these simple gel air fresheners that are scented with our favorite essential oils.

These sweet little fresheners can be used anywhere you would use a store-bought one—in the bathroom, kitchen, laundry room, mudroom, wherever you might have detected an unpleasant scent.

Of course, make sure they stay out of the reach of children and pets. Although most of the ingredients are edible, this recipe does contain a large amount of essential oils for the scent, so it shouldn't be consumed.

Unlike the Deodorizer Disks (page 121), these gel air fresheners don't remove existing unpleasant smells, but they leave a lovely scent in the air.

—————————— WHAT YOU NEED ——————————

30 drops of your favorite essential oils
1½ cups filtered water, divided
3 tablespoons unflavored gelatin
1 tablespoon salt

Choose your container or containers. This recipe will make one air freshener in a 2-cup jar. You will need 30 drops of essential oils for the entire recipe, so if you are making several from one recipe, divide the oils among the containers you are using. The liquid you will be pouring into them will be hot, so you need containers that won't break under heat. I prefer using small glass jelly or mason jars.

The essential oils go in first. In a saucepan on medium heat, warm up 1 cup of water. Whisk in the gelatin until combined. Add the salt and the remaining ½ cup of water and stir just until the salt has dissolved. Pour the liquid into the container or containers with the essential oils. Give a few small stirs to incorporate the oils thoroughly in the liquid.

Let the air fresheners set up (it will take about an hour) and then place in any room. Since they are made with natural ingredients, you will need to replace these air fresheners every 2 to 4 weeks or they can get moldy. For a product that lasts a little longer, you may want to consider the recipe for Deodorizer Disks (page 121).

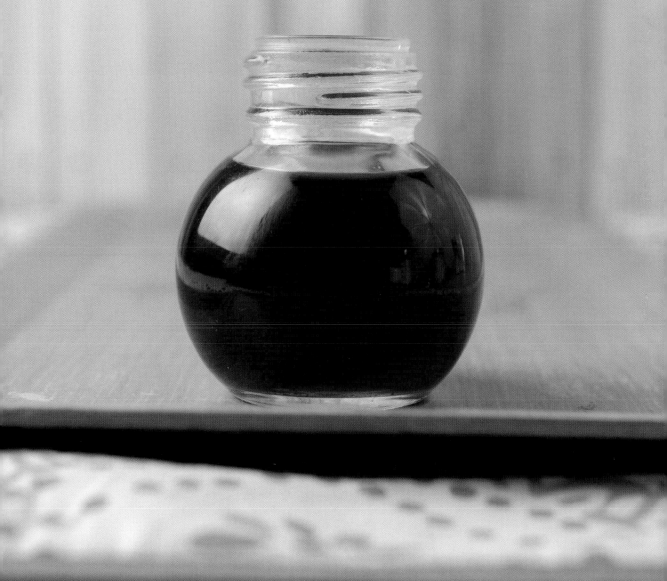

Money-Saving Tip: When it comes to keeping your home smelling fresh, sometimes the best solution is to try to find the root of the problem. Occasionally it's from something that can't be helped (like the trash can or the compost), but often a bad smell is an indication that something is wrong, such as mold under the carpet. Finding and solving the issue might save you money in the long run!

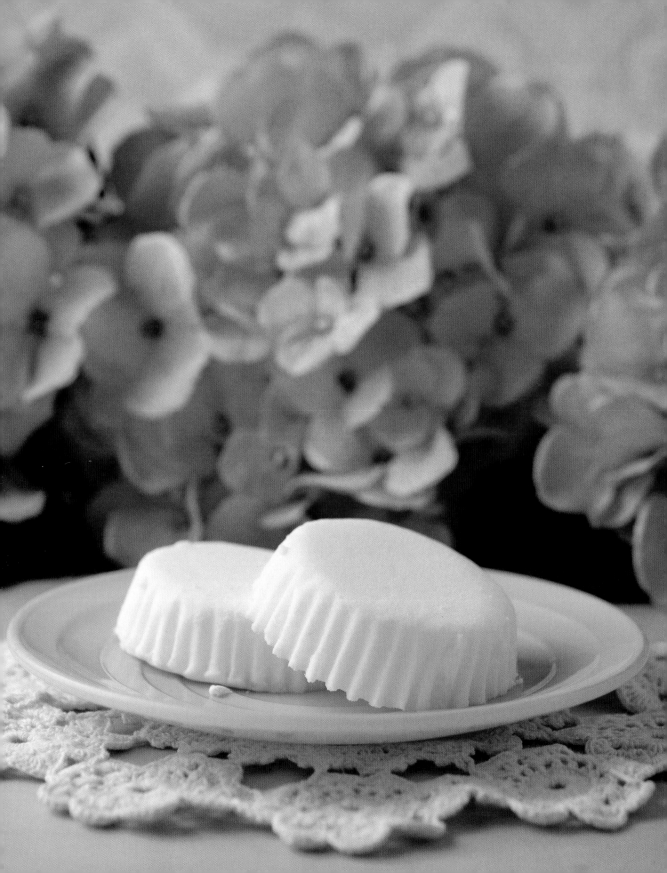

deodorizer disks

. . .

If you have an area of your house that tends to smell like something you don't want it to smell like (like a trash can, fridge, etc.), these little Deodorizer Disks are great to have on hand. You can make these up very quickly and place them anywhere they need to go. And unlike just sprinkling baking soda or another powder in the offending area, these are easy to clean up when they've come to the end of their deodorizing power.

I have several household and craft recipes that use a muffin pan, and since I prefer not to use the same one we use for everyday baking, I have just picked up a spare muffin pan from the dollar store to use for projects like this. It works perfectly! This recipe makes about 9 disks.

WHAT YOU NEED

2 cups baking soda
¾ to 1 cup filtered water
20 drops of your favorite essential oils (optional)

In a bowl, mix together the baking soda and water. Add only enough water to form a thick paste. Once blended to the right consistency, add the essential oils for scent (or leave them out for a simple fragrance-free deodorizer). Pour about ½ inch of the mixture into each cup of a greased or nonstick muffin pan. You can also use muffin liners in the pan to make the disks easy to remove.

Let the disks dry for about a day and remove from the muffin tin. Place anywhere you need a deodorizer. Replace disks after about a month. Store unused disks in a ziplock storage bag or an airtight container until you need them. I make a little note on my daily planner for when I need to replace the deodorizer disks in my trash can and fridge.

Money-Saving Tip: Like vinegar, baking soda is a truly multipurpose product. We usually buy the largest bag that our warehouse store sells, and it's still only around $5. That baking soda can be used for baking, cleaning, and making fun crafts! Skip the tiny boxes and go with the bag next time.

candles and wax melts

· · ·

I love having candles around the house, especially in the winter. The warm glow that each candle casts upon the farmhouse walls makes everything feel more cozy and comfortable. We have candles or the supplies to make them on hand at all times, in case we are in need of some emergency lighting. Here are several kinds of candles that I like to make on a regular basis, depending on what wax or oil I happen to have on hand.

Olive Oil Candles

Olive oil candles have no scent, burn without smoking, and can be made in a hurry if you are in need of some light. Plus they are an excellent way to burn up rancid olive oil. In the book *The Long Winter*, Ma creates a light by using a button, some calico fabric, and some axle grease when she had nothing else. The first olive oil candle I ever made was on a dark winter's night when the power was out and I was stumbling around in the kitchen. Using a flashlight, I grabbed things close to me (olive oil, a jar, a paper clip, and some wick) and rigged up a little candle and we managed to make a nice supper in the dark.

─────────── WHAT YOU NEED ───────────

Thin steel wire (paper clip wire works well)
Candle wick
Mason jar
Olive oil

Using a pair of pliers, create a hook on one end of a small piece of wire (to hook over the edge of the jar). Wrap the other end around a piece of wick. Coil the wire around a piece of wick roughly 4 inches long. Pull about ½ inch of wick out of the coiled wire. Place the hooked end of the wire over the side of the jar so that the wick sits down in the jar.

Take the jar and pour a small amount of oil in the bottom. You can always add more later, so don't feel like you need to make a large candle; just pour in enough to reach to the coiled part of your wire. Don't cover the wick in oil or there won't be anything to burn.

As your candle burns, the wick will draw the olive oil up into itself for fuel. If the flame goes out, you may need to pull up more wick or adjust the wick. Make sure to

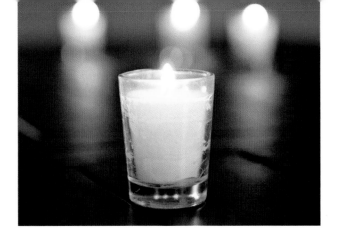

burn this candle on a flat, sturdy surface. For a fresh scent, add a few drops of essential oils or some herbs.

Beeswax Candles

These are one of my favorite candles to make! They last a long time and have a sweet, natural scent. I almost always have beeswax on hand, so we can make these anytime!

The key to making these candles and getting them to work is to add coconut oil to the beeswax. Beeswax is a very hard wax and burns very slowly, so a 100 percent beeswax candle tends to burn through the middle of the candle, leaving you with lots of wasted wax around the edges. Even though this candle will burn a little faster than a pure beeswax candle, you will still need to make sure to get a thicker wick so the candle burns evenly. Each brand of wick has different numbers for different sizes so you may have to experiment with the brand you choose to see which of their wicks will burn best in these candles.

—————— WHAT YOU NEED ——————

Wick (a large, thick wick is needed)
Metal wick holder (optional)
Pint mason jar
1 cup beeswax
1 cup coconut oil (extra-virgin if possible)
10 to 20 drops of your favorite essential oils (optional)

Start by preparing your jar. Use a metal wick holder, which you can buy from the same place you get your wick (or just use a piece of tape), to stick the bottom of your wick in place in the jar. Take the other end of the wick and measure it so it's slightly taller than the jar and cut. Wrap that end around a pencil that can lie across the top of the jar and secure with tape.

In a saucepan, melt the beeswax and coconut oil together over low heat. Add in 10 to 20 drops of essential oils for a naturally scented candle. Slowly pour the mixture into the jar around the wick. Let the candle sit and cool for several hours before trimming the wick ½ inch above the top of the wax.

Money-Saving Tip: Use the wax from leftover candles to make new candles. Leave the candles in a warm place and scrape out the leftover wax. Add to new candles as you are melting the wax. Just make sure, if the candles were scented, that you are adding complementary scents to the new batch.

Other Candle Variations

Soy Candles
Soy candles are very inexpensive to make. When purchased in bulk, you can find soy wax for less than $2 to $3 per pound, whereas beeswax will cost you at least $12 per pound. Soy candles are made using the same method as the beeswax candles above, but instead of beeswax and coconut oil, use only soy wax. Add a few drops of essential oils for some scent in your candle.

Citronella Candles
There is no need to spend extra money on the highly scented citronella candles from the store to keep the mosquitoes off your deck this summer. To create your own, simply add at least 20 to 30 drops of citronella essential oil into either the beeswax candle recipe or the soy candle recipe above.

Wax Melts
You know those expensive little candle melts for candle warmers? You don't really need to buy those! You will only need to invest in some wax tart molds, which are inexpensive and can be purchased online or at craft stores. Then you can either use the soy candle recipe or the beeswax–coconut oil combo to create your wax base. Of course, for wax melts, add several drops of your favorite essential oils, since the main idea behind wax melts is to release scent into the air.

jewelry cleaner

· · ·

I've never been one to have much jewelry, but I do like to wear a nice pair of earrings occasionally. Since I don't bring out my jewelry very often, it tends to get tarnished easily in the humidity of our home.

This jewelry cleaner is so easy and frugal to make, you can whip up a small batch whenever you need to. As with all cleaners, make sure you test on a small area of your jewelry first before cleaning the entire piece. This jewelry cleaner is not for fine silver or gold.

─────────── WHAT YOU NEED ───────────

1 teaspoon toothpaste
1 teaspoon baking soda
½ cup filtered water

Place all the ingredients in a small container and stir to dissolve the toothpaste. Put any jewelry that needs to be cleaned into the container and close the lid (make sure it's on tight). Shake the container for a minute and then let the jewelry soak for another few minutes. Remove the jewelry from the container and wipe off with a dry cloth. The tarnish should come right off. If it doesn't, you may want to scrub the piece with an old toothbrush and let it soak for a while longer before wiping dry again.

Money-Saving Tip: Keep a minimalist jewelry drawer. Only keep jewelry that is either meaningful or something that is multipurpose and can be worn for many different occasions.

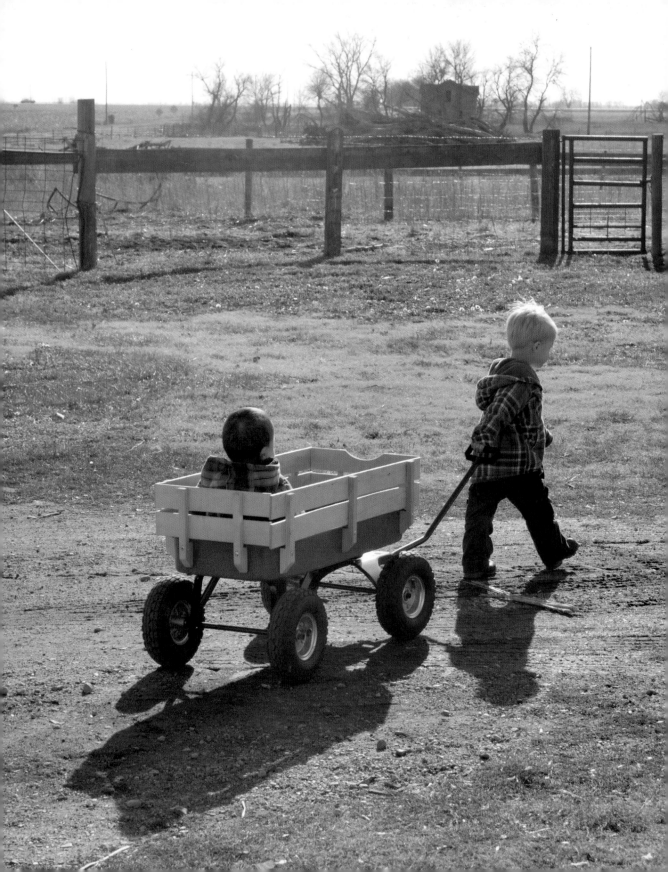

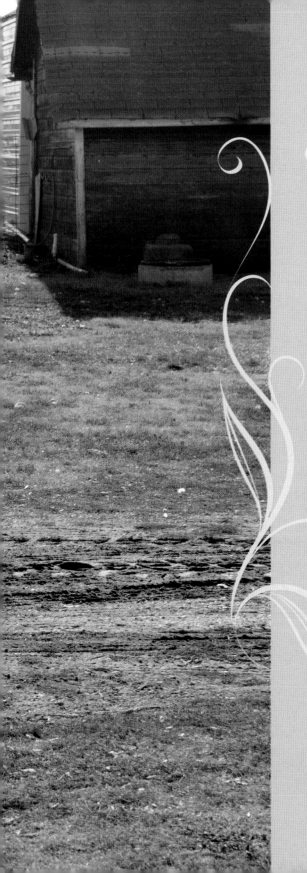

Children
and Pets

*The greatest legacy one can pass on to one's children
and grandchildren is not money or other material
things accumulated in one's life, but rather a legacy of
character and faith.*
—Billy Graham

I remember the time before we had kids. I felt like I'd done all my research and I knew exactly what I wanted to use on my children and I'd make statements such as, "I will never use a disposable diaper!" and "I will never give my children cookies before suppertime!" I think over the years I've learned a valuable lesson . . .

Never say never.

It didn't take long for my "rules" to go right out the window when our first son arrived at our home. In the beginning I used cloth diapers when I could, I fed him healthy foods, and I made sure our house was cleaned up every night before my husband arrived home from work. Then, slowly but surely, my resolve to follow the "rules" started to sneak away. Before I knew it, snack time lasted all afternoon, I went for weeks without using a cloth diaper, and playing in mud puddles became a daily occurrence. When I first realized I'd let myself "slip," I was a little upset. Where were my standards? How would I keep a nice house? What did my husband think I did all day when he came home to this?

I needed to remind myself that this is life, and life is messy. Life isn't perfect. Life isn't black-and-white. And life can be much simpler if we let it go and move with the natural flow of things.

After I realized this I became a much more relaxed mom, and by the time our second son arrived, I'd already heard many comments about how I was so laid-back that they thought I'd been a mom (and had many more children) for a much longer period of time already. The real truth was that I just gave up my view of perfection quicker and realized what the more seasoned moms tend to already know . . . having kids is messy and that's okay.

Our days follow a simple routine. I get up before dawn (and several hours before the family) to have time to myself, time to work, and a bit of time to attend to the house and get meals ready for the day. When they smell breakfast (and my husband smells his coffee), the boys march downstairs ready to start the day. We've started a bit of early homeschooling with our older son, so in the morning he gets some fun but educational activities. Mid-morning, while the baby and I stay inside, he heads outside and watches Daddy work in his shop and fix things around our little farmstead. In the summer we are all outside in the morning and working in the garden. Our goal from year to year is to produce more and more food from the garden to preserve so eventually we won't have to rely much at all on buying produce from the store. The garden is a family project and although the baby is too young to help right now, he loves to sit and watch his brother try to carry a large zucchini from the plant to the wheelbarrow.

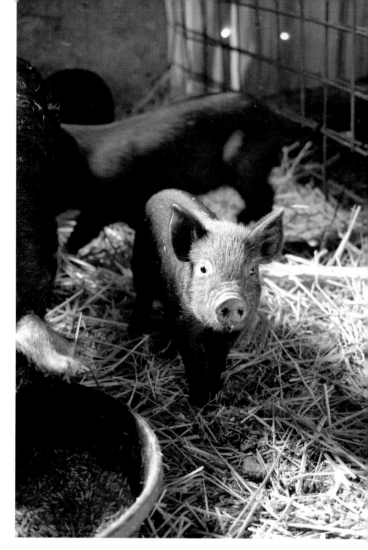

This is the flow of our morning and the basic flow for the rest of the day. We have plenty of work to do to keep up our simple lifestyle, but at the same time, we get to do it together as a family, and the little ones are learning valuable life skills along the way. In the afternoon you can catch us drawing with some of my Rainbow Sidewalk Chalk (page 145) or maybe swinging together in the yard, and in the evening on a nice night we love to take a good family walk down the country roads.

Our lives are messy. Taking care of goats, battling rain to harvest food from the garden, and even using that homemade sidewalk chalk (that somehow tends to end up more on the little ones' skin and clothing than it does on the sidewalk)—all these are messy. But it's nothing a little water (and a little of my homemade Children's Wash, page 132) won't solve.

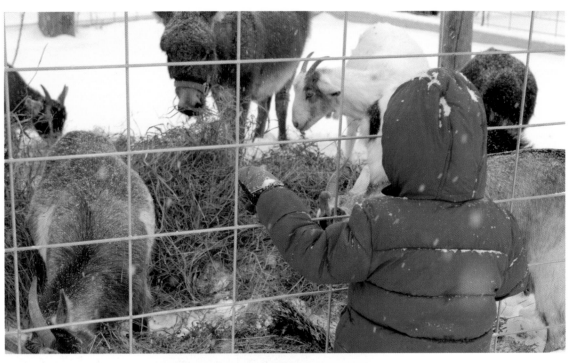

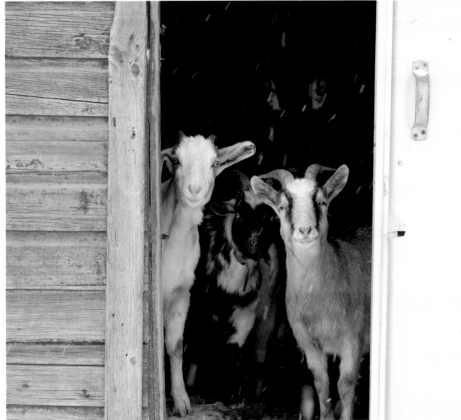

When I was growing up we played in the dirt and in the mud. I specifically remember one year when we built forts out of tumbleweeds underneath some bushy trees. It wasn't clean and it wasn't perfect, but it was beautiful, creative, imaginative play, and I want to give my children the same opportunities to let their imaginations soar.

Our children mean everything to us and we strive to give them the best life possible. Both our little ones have skin troubles, especially our older son, who has multiple food allergies. Even the products that I'd researched and that seemed acceptable to use before we had children had way too many ingredients, and those I tried seemed to cause just as many reactions as any of the other more chemically processed products out there.

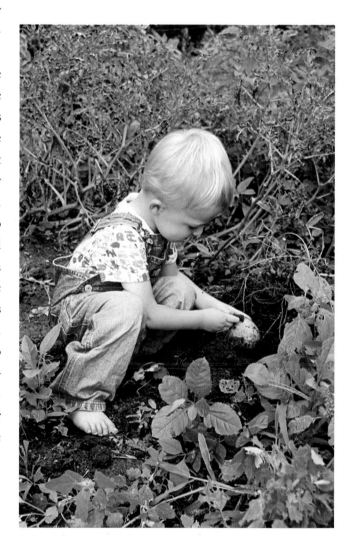

In this chapter you'll find some of my favorite recipes that we've come up with over the last few years of having children. They are simple and use few ingredients and, at least in our case, have proven to be very gentle on those with allergy issues. Not to mention that I don't have to dip into my children's college fund to purchase them! It might sound a little hard to believe, but the recipe that has saved us the most money is our Outdoor Bubbles (page 147). On a nice day, my boys can go through a big container of them— often spilling them in their bubble-blowing excitement—but either way, the container is empty at the end of the day!

children's (mud puddle) wash

. . .

My older boy has a favorite hobby: mud puddles. Big, small, deep, shallow . . . put him in sight of any mud puddle, and he will be there within seconds. We even have special play clothes that I put on him in the morning if I see it rained the night before.

I fully believe any little one should be able to have his fill of mud puddles, so I encourage the dirt, the water, and the mess. The ear-to-ear grin on his little face always makes it totally worth the cleanup.

Speaking of which . . . when he finally comes inside and is ready to be cleaned up, we need something to do it with! I don't use any shampoo or body wash on my babies when they are little; they simply don't need it and water will generally suffice. But once the playing outside and mud puddle phase kicks in, it's time for something that will get my little one squeaky clean again. This recipe, like most of my recipes, is incredibly simple and easy to put together but it gets the job done. I add the oil for an extra moisturizer on my little ones' dry skin, but you are welcome to leave that out if your little one has naturally oily skin. This recipe will work as a body wash or as a shampoo, but keep in mind that it is not "tear-free," so use around little eyes with caution.

─────────── WHAT YOU NEED ───────────

¼ cup castile soap

¾ cup filtered water

1 teaspoon coconut oil (extra-virgin if possible)

Mix all the ingredients together and pour into an old body wash or shampoo bottle. Just give it a little shake before pouring some out so all the ingredients are incorporated. If you find that the mixture is too runny, try putting it in an old foaming hand soap dispenser. It works very well and my little ones love the bubbles!

We use a simple unscented castile soap in this recipe to keep it fragrance-free, and you can use any kind of oil that you have on hand (almond oil, jojoba oil, coconut oil, avocado oil, etc.). And of course, as I mentioned above, you can simply leave out the oil if you feel like your little one doesn't need it.

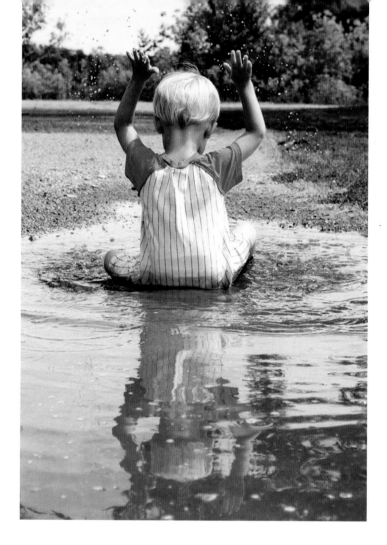

This is a great recipe to make with your little ones because it's so incredibly simple. Have them help you mix together the ingredients or hold the bottle and the funnel while you pour the mixture into its container.

And of course . . . never forget to enjoy the mud puddles.

Money-Saving Tip: Keep one or two outfits for your little ones simply for outside play. That way they don't ruin the nice and everyday clothing you have for them but they can still have fun getting messy!

bubble bath

• • •

What little one doesn't love a good bubble bath after a long day playing? I didn't give the children bubble baths for a very long time, until I found a brand that their skin would tolerate. But you know how much that little tiny bottle was? Sixteen dollars per bottle! Not exactly something that fit into my monthly budget, and we seemed to use up that one bottle very quickly. Instead of enjoying watching my children have fun with the bubbles in the tub, I kept thinking, "Well, there's another two dollars down the drain tonight."

Homemade bubble bath is something that took me a while to figure out. It seems like no matter what I did, it wouldn't bubble up quite like store-bought bubble bath (thanks to all those wonderful chemicals that we really don't want!), and I didn't want it to have a drying effect, since my older son already had very dry skin.

This recipe will definitely produce bubbles and you know exactly what's in it. Not to mention it won't cost you an arm and a leg!

--------- WHAT YOU NEED ---------

½ cup grated bar soap
1 cup filtered water
2 tablespoons vegetable glycerin (food-grade)
1 tablespoon honey (do not use with children under the age of one)
1 tablespoon aloe vera gel

In a saucepan on medium heat, melt the grated bar soap in the water until completely dissolved. Remove from heat and add the vegetable glycerin, honey, and aloe vera. Store in a container in the bathroom until ready to use. Pour under running water to create bubbles in the bathtub. As with any soap, do not let your little ones drink the water.

We use an unscented castile bar soap in this recipe to create a fragrance-free wash. You could use a citrus or peppermint-scented castile soap for something a little different or even your favorite bar soap. (Some of the commercial bar soaps can be very irritating, so make sure to try them on skin first.) Of course, don't forget that both peppermint and citrus are stimulating, so if you plan to use this as a before-bed type of bubble bath, use the unscented wash.

If your little ones are old enough, have them help you grate up the soap bar for this recipe and stir the mixture on the stove while it's melting.

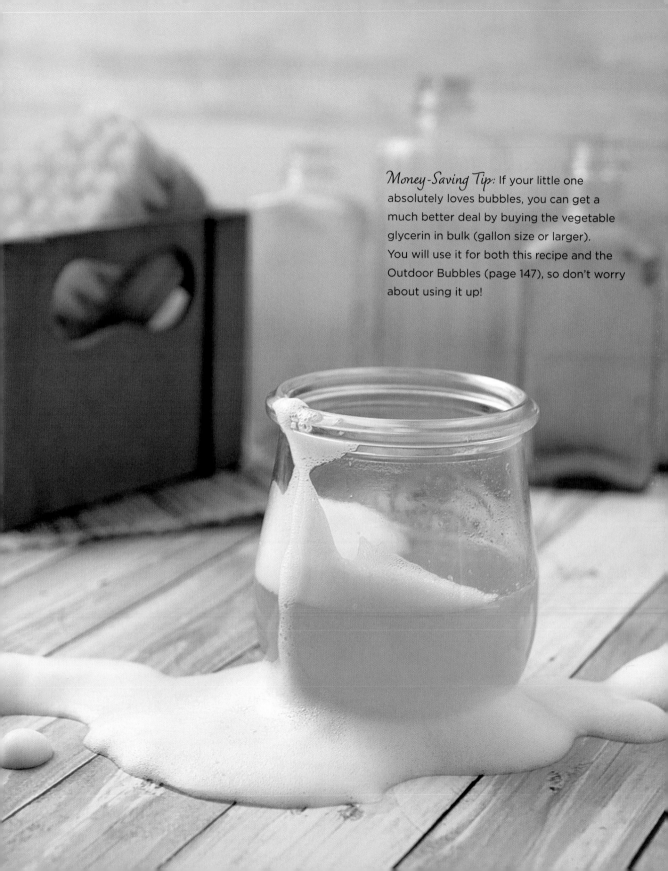

Money-Saving Tip: If your little one absolutely loves bubbles, you can get a much better deal by buying the vegetable glycerin in bulk (gallon size or larger). You will use it for both this recipe and the Outdoor Bubbles (page 147), so don't worry about using it up!

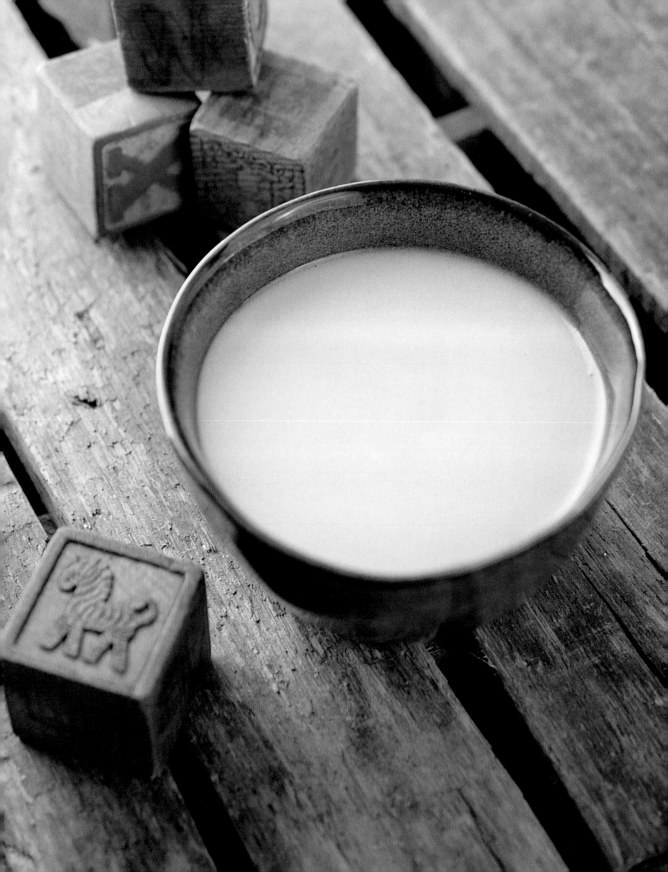

baby lotion

· · ·

There's nothing quite like feeling your new baby's soft skin. It makes you a little bit jealous, doesn't it? Unfortunately, once babies and little ones are introduced to the world, their skin can get dry, flaky, and irritated, just like yours.

Usually when we notice dry skin, we simply rub a little extra-virgin coconut oil into their skin right away to repair it and get it moisturized quickly. However, if the skin is very dry or there are several patches of dry skin, this lotion is very helpful to have on hand. It's very smooth and ultrahydrating and will heal up your little one's dry skin in no time. We generally do not add any essential oils to this recipe, since we use it on babies and because I love the pure, natural scent of babies and wouldn't want a lotion to overpower it! Before long that little one is going to smell like dirt, sweat, and maybe even dog drool, so enjoy it while you can!

———————— WHAT YOU NEED ————————

½ cup mango butter
¼ cup coconut oil (extra-virgin if possible)
1 tablespoon vitamin E oil
¼ cup avocado oil

In a saucepan on medium heat, melt the mango butter and coconut oil together. Pour the mixture into a bowl and add the vitamin E oil and the avocado oil. Beat with an electric hand mixer for a few minutes until smooth and creamy. Place in a jar or container and use when needed. The mixture will harden up slightly as it cools.

Money-Saving Tip: Babies don't need the fanciest and best new baby items on the market. Stick with a crib, blankets, clothing, and bottles to fulfill their basic needs. The regular stroller will get them around in the exact same way as a $500 stroller. And babies go through clothing so fast, if you have too much for them you won't even get to see it all before they move on to the next size!

diaper rash cream

. . .

I remember buying my first tube of diaper rash cream. It was crazy expensive and it didn't work. Not to mention it just felt odd on my fingers and didn't seem like it would be very soothing.

Not long after that experience I came up with this recipe for my own homemade version, and I will tell you right now that it's hands down one of my very favorite DIY recipes ever.

It's simple, soothing, and works incredibly fast. We don't limit the use of this cream to just diaper rash—we use it on any kind of rash! It absorbs well into the skin and heals the rash in no time. As of yet, we have not had any rash that's taken longer than twenty-four hours to look significantly better after applying this cream. It's quite amazing!

As you might imagine, living in the country comes with a variety of rashes that seem to pop up at any time. We've had everything from poison ivy rashes to tomato plant rashes (I'm allergic to the plants!) and this little cream is always the solution. When friends ask me what we use for rashes and I tell them it's my diaper rash cream, they tend to be a little skeptical, but once they've tried it, it's an entirely different story!

WHAT YOU NEED

½ cup shea butter
¼ cup coconut oil (extra-virgin if possible)
1 tablespoon beeswax
2 tablespoons vegetable glycerin

Put the shea butter, coconut oil, and beeswax in a saucepan on medium heat, and stir until melted. Remove from heat and add the vegetable glycerin. Pour the mixture into another bowl and beat until creamy with an electric hand mixer. Pour into a jar or container and let it cool and set up before using. Store in a cool, dry place and use as needed.

This cream is safe for cloth diapers. If you plan on using it with cloth diapers, just make sure to use the ivory shea butter rather than the gold, so it won't leave any yellow stains.

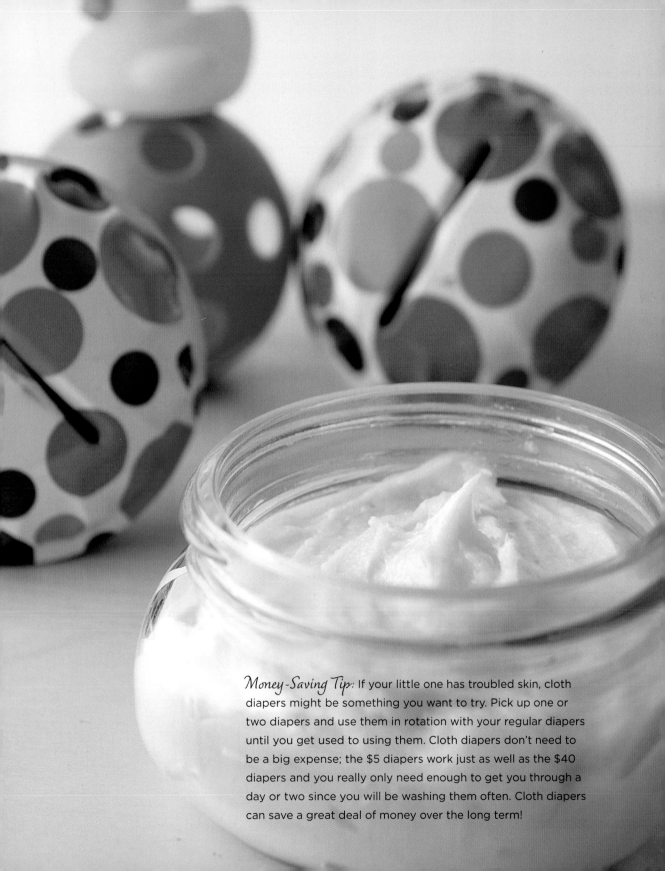

Money-Saving Tip: If your little one has troubled skin, cloth diapers might be something you want to try. Pick up one or two diapers and use them in rotation with your regular diapers until you get used to using them. Cloth diapers don't need to be a big expense; the $5 diapers work just as well as the $40 diapers and you really only need enough to get you through a day or two since you will be washing them often. Cloth diapers can save a great deal of money over the long term!

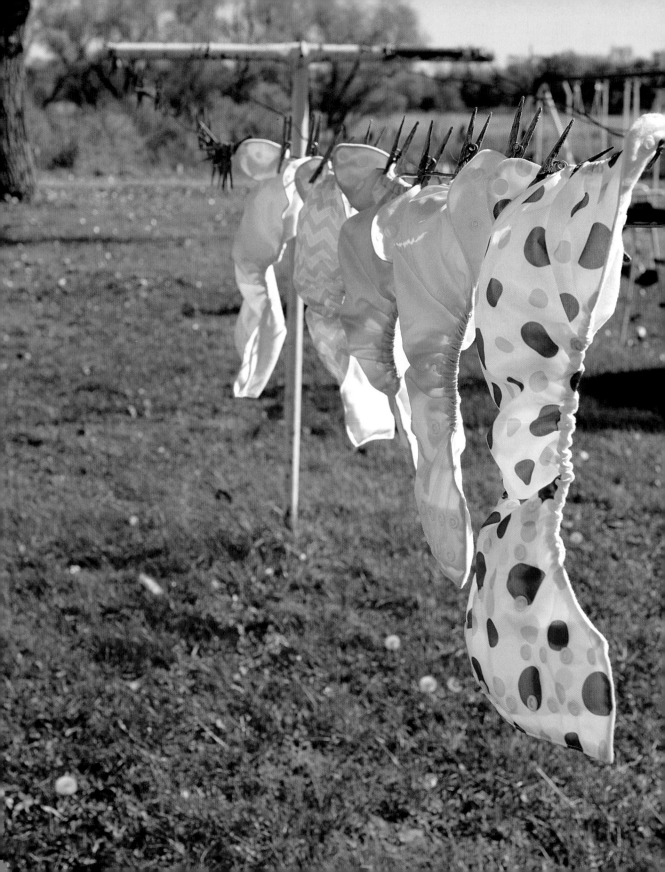

baby wipe solution

. . .

If you make your own baby body products such as diaper rash cream and baby pow-der, it makes perfect sense to make your own baby wipe solution as well! Besides, have you seen some of the ingredients in baby wipes lately? The original idea behind the baby wipe was to get the baby clean and prevent the area from being chafed—I'm just not sure how a chemical concoction is the right solution for that.

You can do one of two things with this solution. Either use it with cloth wipes (which you can make out of flannel or purchase, or just use soft, thin washcloths) or you can make your own disposable wipes with thick paper towels. The most cost-efficient version is the cloth wipes, while the most convenient is the disposable wipes.

Directions for both cloth and disposable versions can be found below. Here's the recipe to get you started.

WHAT YOU NEED

1 cup filtered water

½ cup witch hazel

1 teaspoon aloe vera gel

1 drop lavender essential oil

(optional)

1 drop tea tree essential oil

(optional)

Mix all the ingredients together in a spray bottle. You can leave out the essential oils for a fragrance-free version. Spray the mixture onto wipes before using.

For cloth wipes, simply spray the mixture onto pieces of cotton flannel cloth before using. Keep a pail or wet bag near your diaper-changing area and toss the dirty wipes in after using (you may want to rinse off the full wipes first). Wash the same as you would cloth diapers.

For disposable wipes, remove the cardboard tube from the center of a roll of thicker paper toweling and use a bread knife to cut it in half. (You can skip this step if your roll has half sheets.) You can either spray the paper toweling before using or place the toweling in a bag or container with the solution (so the towels soak it up) so they are ready to be used. Note that pre-moistened towels will not keep as long, so if you are an infrequent wipe user you may want to stick with the spraying method.

Money-Saving Tip: In this case you will want to buy the slightly more expensive paper toweling as it will be thicker and easier to use. You will need less to clean up the mess, so it will actually save you money in the long run.

baby powder

. . .

I'll be honest here: I've never had much of a need to use baby powder on my little ones since any hint of a rash can be cleared up quite quickly with my homemade Diaper Rash Cream (page 138), but my family and friends asked me to create a baby powder recipe for them, so here it is!

─────── **WHAT YOU NEED** ───────

¾ cup arrowroot powder
¼ cup bentonite clay powder
3 drops calendula essential oil (optional)

In a small bowl, mix all the ingredients together. Pour the powder into a sugar shaker for easy use. Adding essential oils to baby powder is optional, and they can be left out for a fragrance-free version. Calendula essential oil is great for baby's skin, but if you can't find it and want to use something you have on hand, lavender oil is a great replacement. We use more arrowroot powder than cornstarch in our home, but again, if you want to use something that is easier to find or that you have on hand, cornstarch will work as a replacement.

If you create this baby powder and find you aren't using it much with the use of your homemade baby wipes and diaper rash cream, there are always other things you can do with it to use it up!

You can use baby powder as a dry shampoo in a pinch. Keep in mind that baby powder would only work for those with lighter-colored hair.

Baby powder can be a great stain releaser on a new stain. Simply sprinkle a very small amount on a clothing stain before washing to help absorb the stain. Launder as usual.

Baby powder is a good foot powder if you want to use something you have on hand without mixing up my Shoe and Foot Spray (page 81). Sprinkle in smelly shoes to help absorb the sweat and the smell.

Freshen up old books (that have that basement mildew smell) by sprinkling a bit of baby powder in the pages and letting them sit for a while. Once the powder has absorbed the smells, brush the powder off.

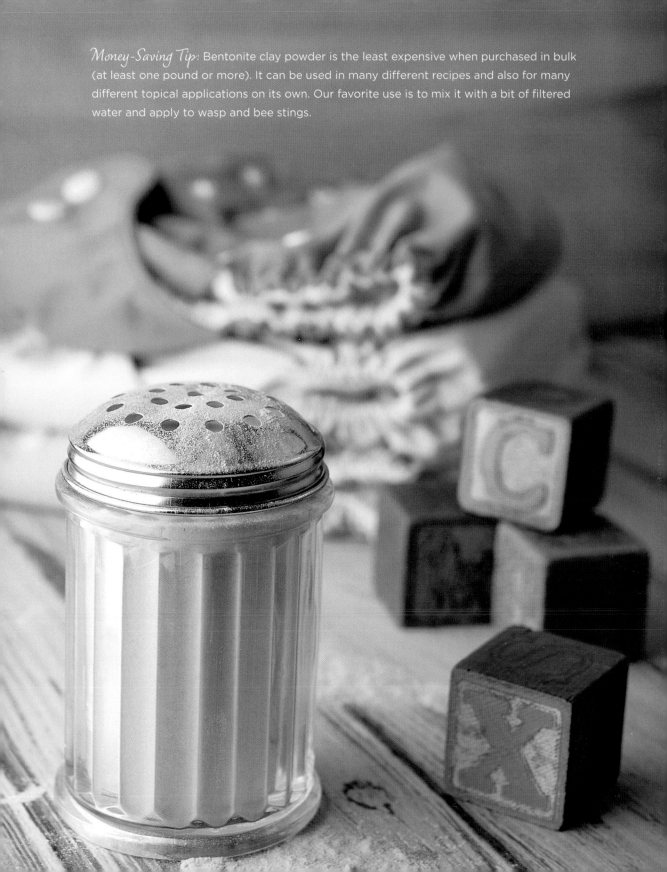

Money-Saving Tip: Bentonite clay powder is the least expensive when purchased in bulk (at least one pound or more). It can be used in many different recipes and also for many different topical applications on its own. Our favorite use is to mix it with a bit of filtered water and apply to wasp and bee stings.

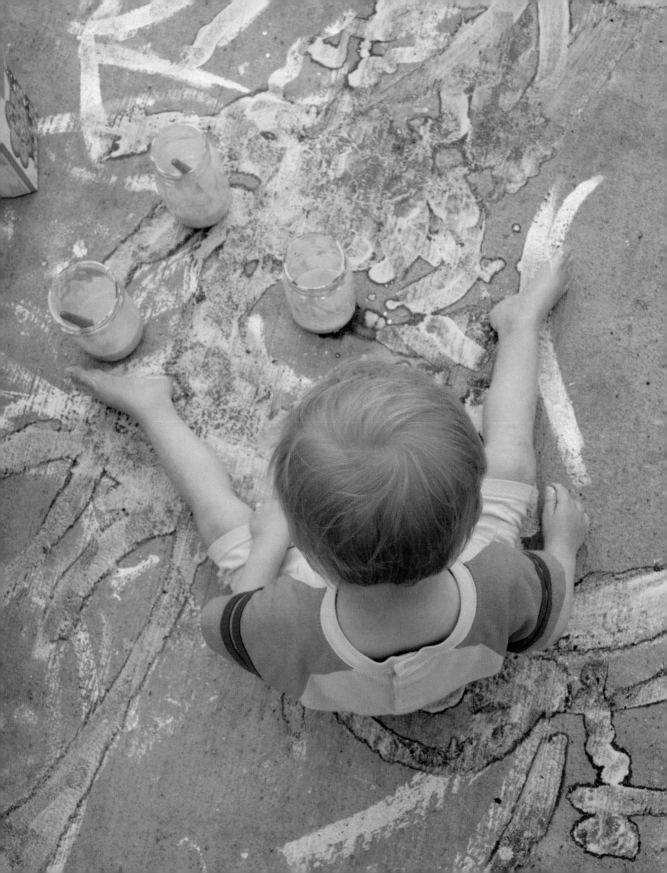

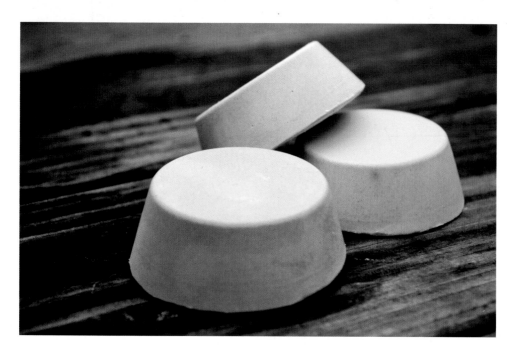

rainbow sidewalk chalk

. . .

I'm always looking for a fun activity for my little toddler, something he can play with on his own with moderate supervision. When we moved into our farmhouse I was excited to see that it had a concrete patio and a small sidewalk, perfect for sidewalk chalk! I was *not* excited when I headed to the store and found that a small container of sidewalk chalk was over $5. And since my toddler is really into tossing sidewalk chalk into puddles . . . I was looking for an inexpensive alternative that wouldn't cost me quite as much to replace.

Sidewalk chalk is very easy to make; just be sure to allow yourself plenty of time to let it dry before you plan to use it. Make it a day ahead, and let it dry overnight. This chalk will wash off the sidewalk or the concrete the same as store-bought sidewalk chalk; just spray with water. I found that these ingredients cost about $8 to make the same amount of chalk that will cost at least $15 or more at the store. Plus this is a great project to create with your children and can even be a color-learning experience.

Any paint will work for this recipe as long as it's labeled "washable." We have found that you can purchase small variety containers of paint, so we never had a lot of extra paint left over that we didn't know what to do with—yet we still had plenty of colors to make several different kinds.

Rainbow Sidewalk Chalk

— WHAT YOU NEED —

½ cup plaster of Paris (dry powder)
½ cup filtered water
1 tablespoon washable paint or food coloring

In a bowl, mix together the plaster of Paris and the water until blended. Add the paint. Don't worry if the mixture doesn't look dark enough after you add the paint; the color will get brighter as the paint incorporates with the plaster.

Pour the chalk into any kind of mold. You can make your own mold out of plastic containers, or if this is something you want to do often, you can purchase a silicone pan for making desserts and treats. It should have forms that are easy for little ones to hold, like stars or flowers. Let the chalk dry overnight before using.

This is a great project to make with your children. Have them help you add the colors into the chalk as you are making it. Share with them the names of the colors or have them tell you the names of the colors as they are adding them. Have them combine a few colors together to show them how color combinations can make new colors.

Money-Saving Tip: Check thrift stores for molds. I almost always see them there for sale as people buy them and then do not really have anything to use them for!

outdoor bubbles

· · ·

You know that feeling you get when you see one of your younger children dressed in a hand-me-down from your oldest?

My first thought is always, "Oh, he is getting so big!" Then my second thought is, "It seems like yesterday when my little Farmer Boy was wearing that same outfit. I mean seriously, was it not yesterday? Wait . . . what day is it today?" Once I get past the confusion, I have a great feeling of sadness. No matter how little my little ones are right now, they are growing and they are certainly growing up fast. It reminds me that my time with them isn't infinite and I want to make sure I take some time to enjoy today.

That's where bubbles come in. You may think they are a little silly and maybe they are an activity that your children could do on their own, but when you make this recipe for homemade bubbles, I hope that you will spend the afternoon sharing the activity with your little ones. Tomorrow is coming too quickly, and before you know it, they will grow out of blowing bubbles with you too.

WHAT YOU NEED

6 cups filtered water

½ cup arrowroot powder

1 tablespoon baking powder

½ cup Dish Soap (page 88)

1 tablespoon vegetable glycerin

In a bucket, mix the water, arrowroot powder, and baking powder until the powders are dissolved in the water. Add the dish soap and glycerin. Do not overstir, because if the bubble mixture starts to foam, it will not produce bubbles and you will need to wait until the foaming goes away to blow bubbles. Use bubble wands (which are reusable) to create big, lovely bubbles with your homemade mixture.

For something fun and different, color some of your bubble mixture with food coloring to make pretty colors. If we plan on doing this, I simply separate some of the bubble mixture from the large jug into a smaller jar and add a few drops of food coloring.

When not in use, store the bubbles in a cool, dark area such as a garage. Warm bubbles simply won't work as well as the cooler version.

Money-Saving Tip: Shop for clothing for little ones out of season. If you are choosing between two sizes to buy, go with the larger size . . . you can always roll up the sleeves or cuffs for a while.

play dough

· · ·

In the winter when the snow and wind are raging outside, it can be hard to find crafts to keep the little ones occupied. We like to find activities that keep them moving and keep their minds busy. I remember when I was growing up, I would simply stare outside and hope that the snow would end quickly so we could head back out and play once again. Apparently this love of the outdoors is something we've already instilled in our children, and it's almost heartbreaking to watch them look out the windows and wish to play outside instead of being stuck in our little house.

Making play dough is a fun activity to break out occasionally. The little ones love to create and "bake" all kinds of goodies to share with Mama. Play dough is very easy to make and there's no need to go to the store for special ingredients; you will find all of these things in your kitchen pantry.

There isn't any need for unnatural dyes; you can simply make it with foods and juices that you already have on hand.

WHAT YOU NEED

1 cup all-purpose flour
(or All-Purpose Gluten-Free Flour
Mix, page 164)
¼ cup salt
2 tablespoons cream of tartar

1 tablespoon olive oil
1 cup filtered water
(colored naturally with one of the
fruits or vegetables listed below)

In a saucepan, combine all the ingredients and mix well. Cook on low heat until the dough starts to pull away from the sides of the pan and form a ball (about 3 to 5 minutes). Allow the dough to cool and place in an airtight container in the fridge to prevent it from drying out. Since the dough has no preservatives, you will want to replace it every few weeks.

Cook these foods in a small amount of water and then use the naturally colored juices to color your play dough.

- Pink or red: red cabbage, strawberries, or raspberries
- Yellow: lemon peels
- Orange: carrots

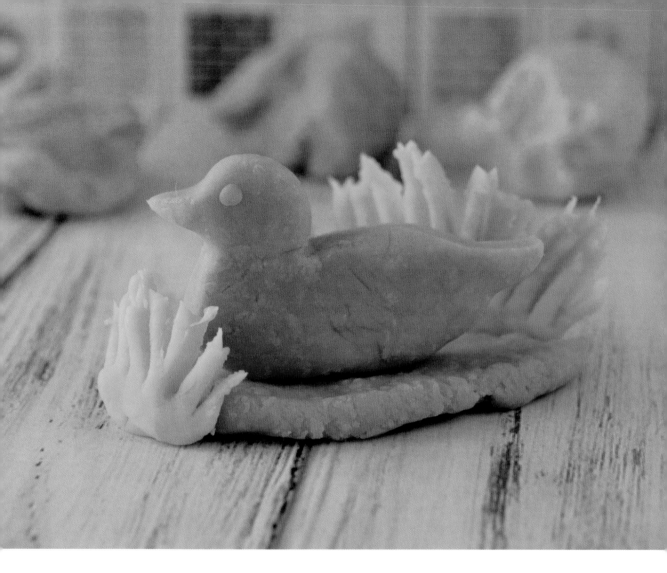

- Blue: blueberries
- Green: spinach

This is another great recipe to get the kids involved. Have them find things around the kitchen that they think would make great colors for their homemade play dough.

Money-Saving Tip: Another fun, indoor sensory-type activity is play sand. In a small storage container, mix together 2 cups flour with ¼ cup melted coconut oil. Once the ingredients are blended, it will feel just like sand and little ones will love to run their fingers through it, draw in it, and use little cups and bowls to shape and play with it.

air-drying clay

· · ·

Sometimes it's fun to take our homemade creations and make them into something that can be kept longer than a simple play dough sculpture. For these kinds of crafts we love to use a homemade air-drying clay. It's easy to sculpt with and is extraspecial because we get to keep the finished product.

We like to use this air-drying clay to make special presents for Grandma and Grandpa. For an extra project, paint the dried products with homemade paint (see pages 151–153). This clay works well to make fun little handprint or footprint memories. I will never forget the first Father's Day we ever celebrated. It was a few months after our older son was born and I wanted to have something special that the baby and I could "make." I simply mixed up some of this clay, formed it into a heart shape, and pressed our tiny baby's feet into it. My husband was touched by the special gift and of course we still have it now as a sweet memory of those tiny little feet.

--------------- WHAT YOU NEED ---------------

2 cups flour	¾ cup filtered water
1 cup salt	2 tablespoons olive oil

In a medium bowl, mix all the ingredients together until incorporated. Knead with your hands until the dough becomes smooth. Store in an airtight container until ready to use. It will only store for a few days, so plan to use it quickly.

Once you've created something with the dough, simply let it dry undisturbed in a warm, dry place for several days. If the creation is thick, you may want to speed the drying process along by placing the item in the oven at a low temp (around 180 degrees) for about 10 minutes.

You can mix things into your dough (special coloring, glitter, etc.) or just leave it plain and paint it when the creation is dry.

Money-Saving Tip: I love looking for crafty items at local garage sales. Often older folks will clean out a craft room and sell large amounts of crafting supplies in bags or boxes. Even an assortment of items can be used for creative children's crafts, and they will cost you much less than you would pay at the craft supply store.

watercolor paints

. . .

I love making homemade watercolor paints. The children seem to love getting to use a paintbrush, and Mama loves to paint with them. This is another recipe that is great to make on a rainy or snowy day because you already have all the ingredients in your pantry. This recipe can use food coloring or you can replace the water with naturally dyed water. (Ideas can be found in the homemade Play Dough recipe, page 148.) We find that this paint is best used on a thicker paper, such as card stock or construction paper. It will easily wash off tables if your little one gets a little *too* artistic.

————————— WHAT YOU NEED —————————

1 cup baking soda
¾ cup white vinegar
2 tablespoons vegetable glycerin
1 cup cornstarch
Food coloring (or colored water)

In a bowl, mix together the baking soda and vinegar. Make sure to add the vinegar very slowly or it may bubble over the bowl and make a mess. Whisk together. Add the vegetable glycerin and the cornstarch. Whisk well until combined.

Using an empty (and clean) ice cube tray, pour small amounts of the paint base into each cavity. Add a bit of coloring to each pocket and mix carefully until the color is even.

Note: If you are using colored water, your paints will not dry out and will need to be used right away.

Let the paints dry in the trays (at least 24 hours). To use, simply add a bit of water on the end of your paintbrush to pick up the paint.

Money-Saving Tip: If your little one is really little, you can skip the paint altogether and still give them the joy of painting. Use colored construction paper and simply give them a paintbrush and a bit of water to dip it in. They can then "paint" the water over the construction paper and of course the paper will turn darker in the spots that they've painted in. It's a great way to teach them how to use a paintbrush without the mess!

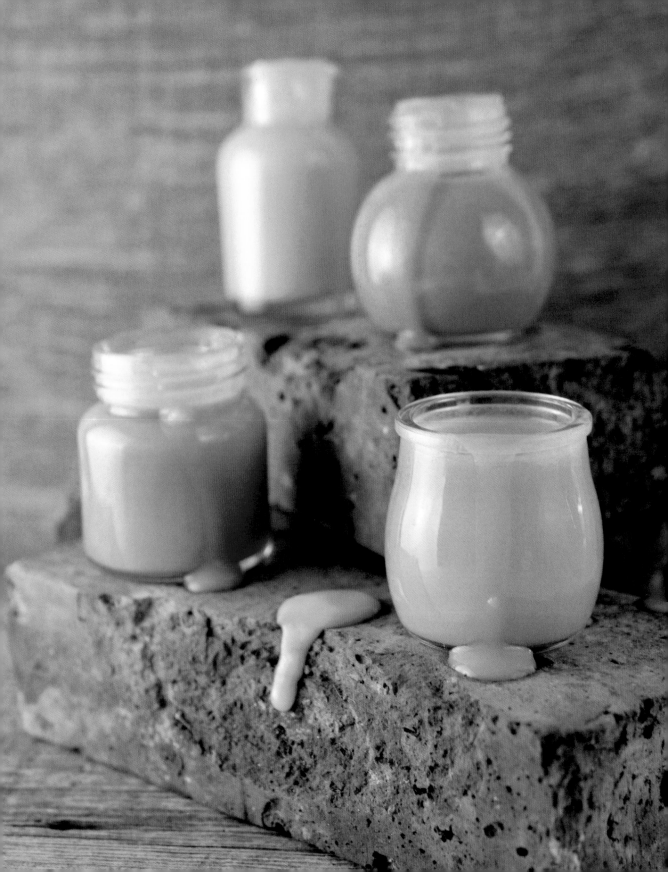

finger paints

· · ·

At our house we happen to think that finger painting is fun for any age. Pretty pictures? Check! Messy fun? Check! It's a great indoor project for when the weather outside is less than perfect and when we want the creativity to flow. You can make finger paints with simple items found in your kitchen pantry. For coloring, you can follow the natural dye ideas for homemade Play Dough (page 148) or you can use natural food coloring.

These finger paints will wash off fingers easily. If your child is gluten-free, replace the regular flour in this recipe with an all-purpose gluten-free blend. It's not something they need to eat, but at least you can feel safe knowing that if a finger finds its way into a mouth, your little one will be all right.

WHAT YOU NEED

1 cup flour
2¾ cups colored filtered water
2 tablespoons salt

If you want several different colors, make sure to make separate, smaller batches of paint. In a saucepan, mix all the ingredients together. Stir with a whisk over low to medium heat until the mixture begins to thicken. Remove from heat and let it cool completely before using. Store in an airtight container in the refrigerator until ready to use. Since this paint uses only natural ingredients, you will want to use it up within a few weeks of making it.

Money-Saving Tip: Old food jars are a perfect way to store paints, craft supplies, and other fun items. Save everything from baby food jars to old salsa jars to have a variety of sizes.

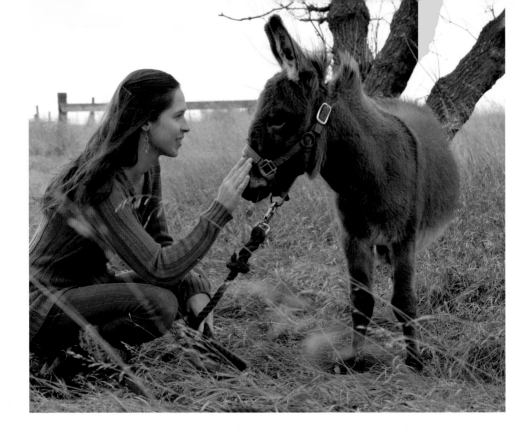

pet shampoo

· · ·

Why is it that our pets love to get into the smelliest things? They'll find something rancid, roll around in it for a while, and then come and show us their new perfume, like we should be proud of them for their accomplishment. Not all of you may have had this experience, but one of the worst things that our pets have done is discover the baby calf pen. Something attracts them to the area, and once they've found it they will bring us all kinds of "treats" and smell less than wonderful all the time.

It's a good thing we haven't yet invented books that you can smell, isn't it? Although I'm guessing your mind is giving you quite the vision right now, so let's move on!

Keeping your pets clean can be a challenge, but it doesn't have to be an expensive one. While a bottle of pet shampoo at the specialty pet stores can cost anywhere from $5 to $20 (or more), this recipe can be made for around $2 for the entire bottle. It will leave your pets clean and smelling fresh and it can be made up pretty quickly, just in case you need it in a hurry.

—————————— WHAT YOU NEED ——————————

1 cup castile soap
2 teaspoons baking soda
1 cup filtered water
5 drops rosemary essential oil
1 tablespoon Dish Soap (page 88)

In a small bowl, mix all the ingredients together. Pour into an old shampoo or lotion container to store and use to wash your pets as needed. Wet your pet, rub in the soap, and wash out thoroughly. For pets with very dry skin, add ¼ cup oat flour or blend ¼ cup uncooked old-fashioned oats in the blender until they become a powder and add them to the mixture. If your pet has extremely dry and flaky skin, add the oats and 1 teaspoon aloe vera gel as well.

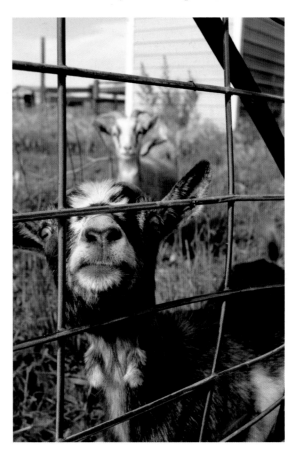

Rosemary essential oil should be safe to use on both cats and dogs, but if your pet has had a reaction to it in the past or is sensitive, you may just want to leave it out.

Money-Saving Tip: Call a vet before you take an animal into the vet's office. If you have a great vet, they may just be able to give you the advice you need over the phone without having to see the animal, saving you an expensive visit.

pet flea wash

. . .

There's something that no pet parent ever wants to deal with but, as with just about anything . . . some things are inevitable, and when they happen, they just need to be dealt with. If your pets are frequently in an area where they might be exposed to fleas, you may want to use this wash on them to help prevent those little creatures from entering your yard and home.

WHAT YOU NEED

1 cup vinegar
1 cup warm filtered water
2 tablespoons Dish Soap (page 88)
1 teaspoon salt
10 drops rosemary essential oil

Mix all the ingredients together in a medium bowl and stir until the salt has dissolved into the mixture. Use as a rinse for your pets to help prevent fleas in their fur and on their bodies. Wet your pet's body, use this wash, and then rinse lightly with water. The addition of vinegar in this recipe can sometimes be drying to a pet's skin, so you may want to add the oats and aloe vera to their next wash.

If you do have fleas in your home or your yard, you can use diatomaceous earth to help remove them. Sprinkle food-grade diatomaceous earth into your carpet or around your yard. Let it sit for a while and then vacuum up any sprinkled into your carpet. The diatomaceous earth is like glass in the fleas' bodies when they eat it and should kill them upon consumption. Look for food-grade diatomaceous earth at your local garden supply stores.

You can also prevent fleas (and some other pet pests) by adding a few drops of tea tree essential oil to your dog's collar. Do not use tea tree oil on cats.

Money-Saving Tip: If you have a feed store in your town, call to see if they sell pet food. Often many feed stores or even grain elevators sell high-quality pet food in bulk so it's much more affordable than your average big-box store. Store excess pet food in clean, new plastic garbage cans with lids.

pet treat mix

· · ·

Every once in a while your pup needs a treat too. And of course, if you plan on making those treats at home, it will be much less time-consuming for you if you already have a mix ready to go.

You should be able to find a cute little bone-shaped cookie cutter to make these treats, but any cookie cutter will do. All the ingredients are human friendly, so you don't need to worry about having special cookie cutters or supplies just for making these treats.

This mix recipe is also a fun thing to give as a gift to your dog-loving friends. When I give this as a gift, I also include the can of pureed pumpkin in the recipe and put it in a little basket along with a cute cookie cutter.

If your dog is in need of a grain-free treat, you can replace the regular flour in this recipe with a grain-free flour such as garbanzo bean flour.

Dog Treat Mix

WHAT YOU NEED

1 cup uncooked old-fashioned oats
½ cup cornmeal
2½ cups all-purpose flour

Mix all the ingredients together and place in a jar or storage bag.

Dog Treats

WHAT YOU NEED

1 jar Dog Treat Mix
1½ cups warm filtered water
1 egg

⅓ cup coconut oil
(extra-virgin if possible)
2 cups pureed pumpkin

In a large bowl, combine the treat mix and the warm water. Add the egg, coconut oil, and pumpkin and mix until all the ingredients are blended. Pour the batter into a greased 9x13-inch baking dish. Bake at 325 degrees for 35 minutes. Cool before letting your pup enjoy. After baking, you can use cookie cutters to cut fun shapes out if you wish or you can simply score the treats into squares that are the perfect size for

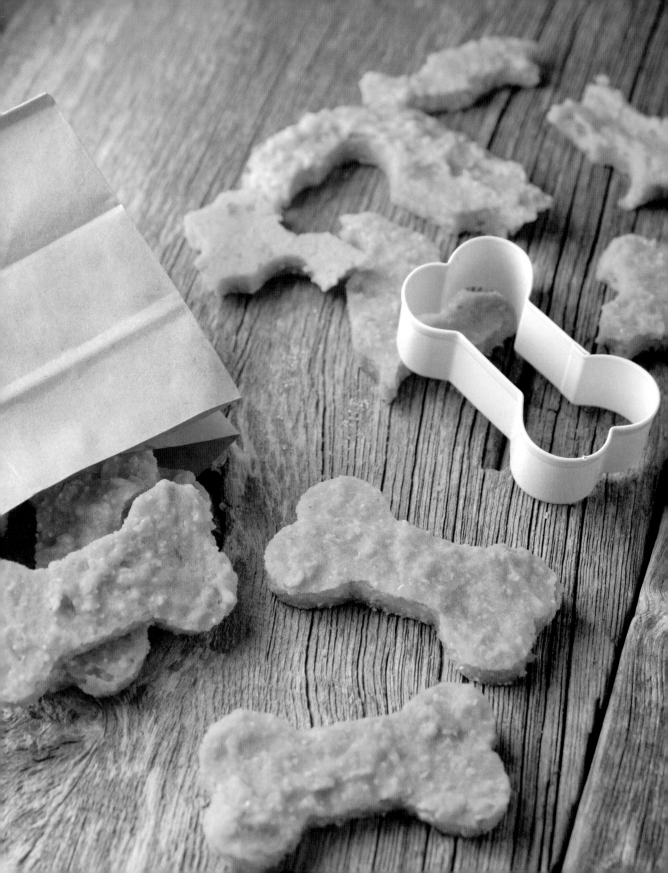

your pet to enjoy. Store these treats in the fridge and use within a week or two. Goats love these for a treat too!

Cat Treat Mix

Cat Treats don't have a large base of dry ingredients, but you can still put together a mix to make it less time-consuming to create when you need them.

─────── WHAT YOU NEED ───────

1 cup all-purpose flour
⅓ cup cornmeal
1 tablespoon coconut oil (extra-virgin if possible)

Mix all the ingredients together and store in a jar until ready to make.

Cat Treats

─────── WHAT YOU NEED ───────

1 jar Cat Treat Mix
1 cup cooked, shredded chicken
½ cup chicken stock

Mix all the ingredients together to form a dough. Roll out onto a lightly greased cookie sheet until the dough is very thin. Cut the treats using a knife or pizza cutter so they are small, treat size. Bake at 350 degrees for 20 minutes. You can replace the chicken with tuna and tuna "juice" for the chicken stock if your cat prefers a tuna-flavored treat.

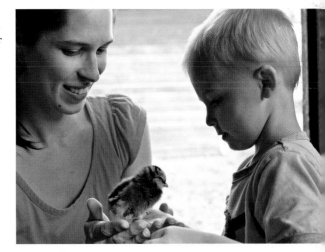

Money-Saving Tip: Make sure you have your pets as part of your monthly budget expenses so you know you have enough to provide for them. We set aside a small amount monthly from our income that is saved specifically for pets' needs.

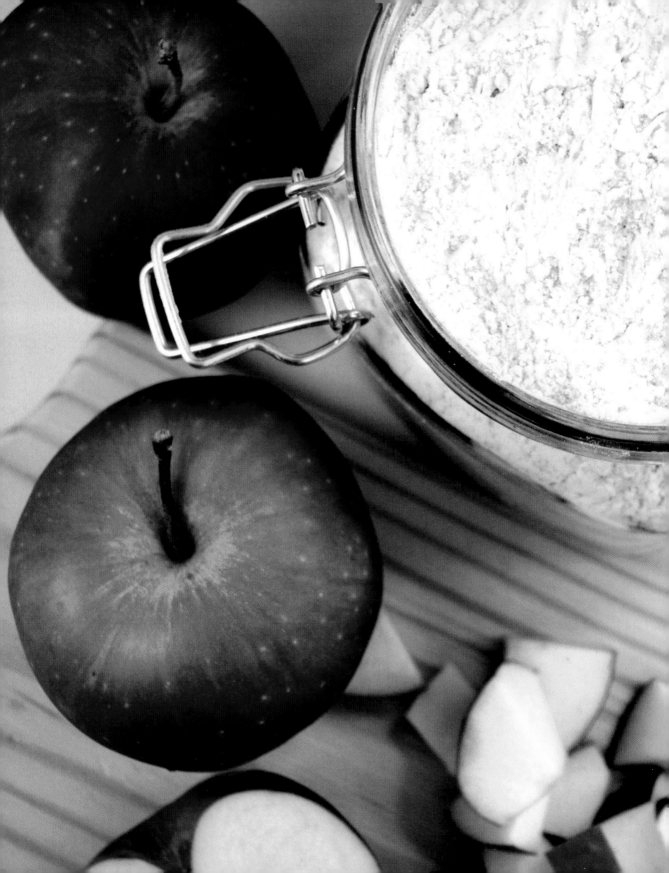

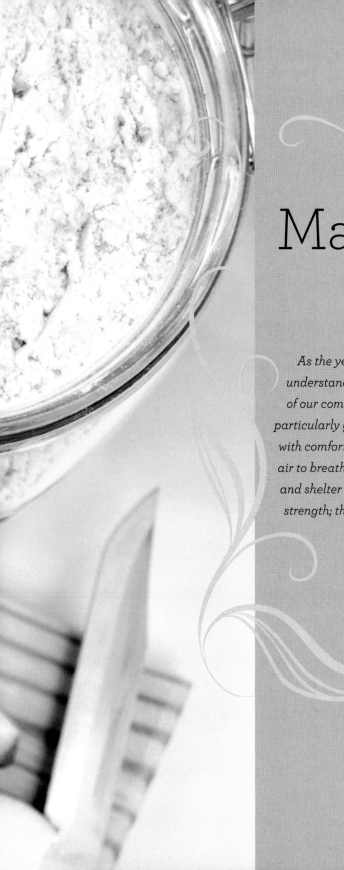

Make-Ahead Mixes

As the years pass, I am coming more and more to understand that it is the common, everyday blessings of our common, everyday lives for which we should be particularly grateful. They are the things that fill our lives with comfort and our hearts with gladness—just the pure air to breathe and the strength to breathe it; just warmth and shelter and home folks; just plain food that gives us strength; the bright sunshine on a cold day; and a cool breeze when the day is warm.

—Laura Ingalls Wilder

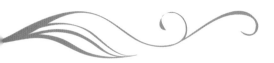

I love food and I love baking, so when I discovered I had food allergies and intolerances, I had no idea what I was going to do or what recipes I would still be able to make. Prior to my diagnosis we ate most of the foods of a typical American diet and unfortunately, much of it was boxed, canned, and pretty expensive.

Over the years I've taught myself to create recipes that I can not only eat, but that are from scratch, can be made in a hurry, and are still delicious!

I love to go to the grocery store and just look at the shelves, not to buy things but to check out the new creative products that are available. When I find something that I think we would like, I take a look at the ingredients and start to put together a picture of how I could make the recipe at home with what I have, or maybe even put together my own "convenience mix" to have in the pantry.

Another big source of inspiration for my recipes is either a family recipe that I'm trying to make to fit in our current lifestyle or an old-fashioned recipe that I found in an old cookbook or tucked away in a recipe card box. Many old-fashioned recipes from way "back in the day" (and I don't mean the '60s; I'm taking about the 1920s or earlier) were made with average, everyday ingredients and not brand-name or "newfangled" ingredients. For this reason, out of my collection of cookbooks, the number of books that are pre-1920s is the largest because the recipes come the closest to things that we like to eat!

Having mixes and premade seasonings in my kitchen pantry saves me a great deal of time when it comes to food prep, not to mention they also create less of a mess while I'm baking, and when you have a tiny kitchen like mine, less mess is ALWAYS a good thing!

By tiny I don't mean just that we don't have a kitchen island (well, we don't, but . . .) and that there's less counter space, I mean that I can literally touch both sides of the kitchen with my arms outstretched. It means that we had to find a tiny fridge because a regular one just wouldn't fit. Originally my kitchen was the pantry in our 1890 farmhouse and was renovated into the kitchen in the 1930s when the house got indoor plumbing and the owners turned what was then the kitchen into the dining room. At our previous house I had a decent-size kitchen with full-size appliances (including a dishwasher!) but somehow I don't miss having that extra space in the farmhouse. I've learned to downsize my kitchen tools and appliances to have only what we really use and really need. So if you come to my house looking for some specialty bar pan for some fancy-shaped brownies, I won't have it, but I will have a regular bar pan that works perfectly fine for brownies. (And the brownies will taste just the same, I promise!) It's fun to have special things when you have the space for them, but if you don't, nothing life-shattering will happen to your cooking. A good supply of the basics is really all you need.

My pantry is put together in the same way that my kitchen is, with simple, basic foods and ingredients.

Speaking of basics, here's a list of things that I always have in my simple pantry:

Baking powder	Dried beans (pinto, black,	Potato starch
Baking soda	and navy)	Raisins
Brown rice flour	Dried tomatoes	Raw honey
Brown rice pasta	Garlic powder	Raw sugar
Chocolate chips	Golden flaxseed	Rice
Cocoa powder	Minced onion	Rice milk
Coconut milk	Oats (old-fashioned and	Sea salt
Coconut oil	quick-cooking)	Unbleached wheat flour
(extra-virgin if	Olive oil	Unflavored gelatin
possible)	Popcorn	

Those are just the basics for our pantry staples. They are the foods I try to keep in stock at all times, because with them I can make just about anything! Along with these basics we also have a healthy supply of our own home-canned goods: fruits like pears, peaches, preserves, and veggies like green beans, corn, and more.

Since we make all our food from scratch, I love making mixes and seasonings to have on my pantry shelves. I still have the convenience benefits of a store-bought mix, but I know all the ingredients in the mix and can control what we can and can't have due to our allergy needs and based on what I have on hand at the time.

By having mixes on hand we can avoid any impulse purchases when we aren't feeling like cooking much or don't have the time, and it makes it much easier to see what I can make based on what I already have in my pantry, which makes weekly meal planning a breeze!

In this chapter you will find some of our favorite basic mixes and seasonings. It's a wide variety of everything from drink mixes (pages 216–219) to a homemade Spanish Rice Mix (page 176). I hope that by using the recipes you will also be able to create delicious home-cooked meals for your family and maybe even feel inspired to start creating some mixes of your very own based on your family's favorite meals and treats.

If stored in airtight containers, these mixes will keep for several months. You can store them for an even longer amount of time by placing them in freezer bags and storing them in the freezer until you are ready to use them.

Note: These recipes will feed a family of four.

All-Purpose Gluten-Free Flour Mix

Since we have gluten allergies in our household, you will notice that the recipes that follow can be made with regular flour or gluten-free flour. Over the years I've created this basic gluten-free flour mixture that is inexpensive and works great in our recipes. My basic recipe does not contain a binding ingredient (such as guar gum), so if you need that in the recipe, you will have to add it in. As a general rule you will need about 1 teaspoon of a binding agent for every cup of flour used in the recipe. You may find with some recipes that contain eggs, bananas, applesauce, or other natural binding agents that you may not need it.

What You Need
    2 cups brown rice flour
    2 cups sweet rice or sticky rice flour
        (you can use coconut flour instead)
    1 cup potato starch
Mix all the ingredients together and store in an airtight container. Use as a cup-for-cup replacement for regular flour in a recipe.

Egg Replacer

If for any reason you need to replace eggs in a baking recipe, there are a few options. In most gluten-free recipes (or regular flour recipes), we replace each egg with 1 tablespoon ground flaxseed and 3 tablespoons filtered water. (Mix those two ingredients together and let them sit for a few minutes before adding to a recipe. Double for 2 eggs, triple for 3 eggs.) In other recipes you can usually replace the egg with ¼ cup vegetable oil, ¼ cup applesauce, or a single mashed banana.

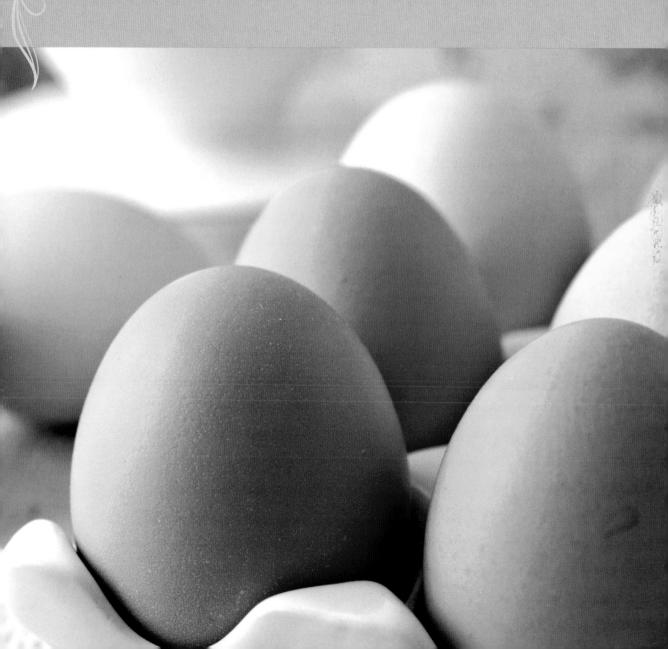

Saving Time Making Mixes

When I refill my pantry with these homemade mixes, there are two different methods I use to save time in the kitchen. One way to fill up your pantry with homemade mixes is to simply make extras of the product while you are making it. So, for example, if you are mixing up a batch of cookies, instead of making one batch just to eat right now, fill a few jars of the cookie mix while you have all the ingredients out. No extra effort and very little extra time is put into doing this and you'll create a few extra mixes to work on filling your pantry just as you go about your everyday life.

Another option is to have a mix-making day. If you have a morning to spare, you can make a large amount of mixes to fill up your pantry. Since many take similar ingredients (flour, sugar, baking powder, etc.) it's easy to mix up many different things at once when you take out all your ingredients and have them on the counter. This method takes a bit more time but you can produce a large amount of mixes to fill up your pantry rather quickly.

Either way you choose to do it, it will work out great because in the end you are able to have a pantry full of delicious mixes and meals. So, without further ado, let's get to it!

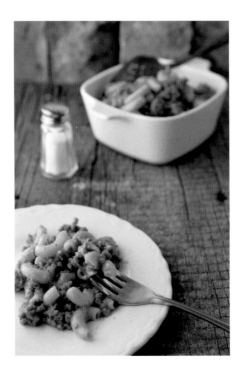

hamburger help mix

· · ·

You know that boxed pasta mix that you buy at the store to go with beef, chicken, or even tuna? Yes, you know what I mean . . . I call it the idea box.

Basically, it takes something boring (meat) and adds flavors and extras to make it one simple meal that's easy to make and perfect for the nights when you feel uninspired to make supper. Plus, I love that it's a "one dish" meal. Less cleanup!

We have something like that at our house too, but we don't buy it from the store; it comes right out of my pantry. It's cheaper to make than the boxed version and I can put together more of it at any time. Keep a few jars of this in your own pantry for quick, easy-to-throw-together meals when you need them.

WHAT YOU NEED

1 tablespoon cornstarch or arrowroot powder

2 teaspoons paprika

1 teaspoon garlic powder

1 teaspoon onion powder

1 teaspoon salt

1 teaspoon sugar

1½ cups uncooked elbow macaroni

Stir all the ingredients together in a bowl until the spices are blended, then pour into a jar or bag. This recipe will fit into a pint-size mason jar or a quart storage bag.

Hamburger Help

WHAT YOU NEED

1 pound ground beef

1 recipe Hamburger Help Mix

2 cups milk

1 cup filtered water

1 cup shredded cheddar cheese

When you are ready to make a meal, brown the ground beef in a skillet. Add the mix into the skillet and pour in the milk and water. Simmer until pasta is cooked through. Stir in shredded cheddar cheese just before serving.

For a chili cheese version, add 1 tablespoon chili powder to the mix.

For a gluten-free version, use gluten-free pasta.

For a dairy-free version, use 2 cups chicken or beef broth in place of the milk and either skip the cheese or use your favorite cheese replacement.

beef stroganoff mix

· · ·

—————— WHAT YOU NEED ——————

2 cups uncooked egg noodles	¼ teaspoon black pepper
1 tablespoon cornstarch or arrowroot powder	1 teaspoon dried parsley (optional)
2 teaspoons paprika	1 teaspoon garlic powder
1 teaspoon salt	1 teaspoon minced onion

Mix all the ingredients together in a bowl until the spices are blended, then pour into a bag or jar.

Beef Stroganoff

—————— WHAT YOU NEED ——————

1 pound ground beef

1 cup chopped fresh mushrooms

1 recipe Beef Stroganoff Mix

2 cups milk or beef broth or stock

½ cup sour cream

Brown the ground beef in a skillet. Add the chopped fresh mushrooms and cook until mushrooms are browned as well. Pour the mix into the skillet and add the milk or beef stock. Let the mixture simmer until the pasta is cooked through. Add the sour cream just before serving.

For a gluten-free version, use gluten-free pasta.

For a dairy-free version, skip the sour cream and use chicken or beef broth instead of milk.

chicken help mix

· · ·

½ teaspoon celery seed

1 tablespoon minced onion

½ teaspoon minced garlic

1 teaspoon sugar

1 teaspoon chili powder

1 teaspoon salt

2 cups uncooked bow tie pasta

Mix all the ingredients together in a bowl until the spices are combined. Store in a jar or storage bag.

Chicken Help

WHAT YOU NEED

1 cup cooked, shredded chicken

1 recipe Chicken Help Mix

1 cup milk

1 cup chicken broth or stock

2 cups (16 ounces) diced tomatoes

Parmesan cheese

In a skillet on medium heat, add the shredded chicken, the mix, the milk, the chicken broth, and the diced tomatoes. Simmer until the pasta is cooked through. Top with a bit of Parmesan cheese before serving.

For a different taste, leave the chili powder out of the mix and add 1 cup shredded cheddar cheese right before serving.

For a gluten-free version, use gluten-free pasta.

For a dairy-free version, skip the Parmesan cheese and add an extra cup of chicken broth instead of the milk.

Money-Saving Tip: Not buying your meat in bulk? If you have the space, the time is now! Look for a rancher who sells meat by the quarter, half, or whole and find out the price per pound and learn how the animals were raised. You can usually get much better deals on much fresher and higher-quality meat than you could ever get at the grocery store.

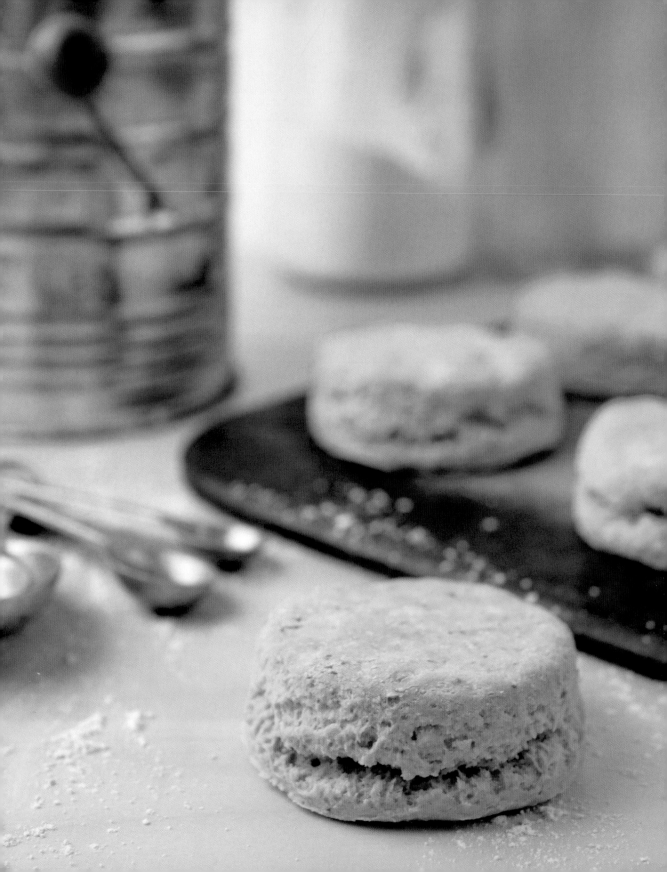

all-purpose baking mix

. . .

One good staple that every kitchen should have is a basic all-purpose baking mix. This mix can be used in many different recipes and it's great to have on hand for when you need to whip up something bready in a hurry.

My All-Purpose Baking Mix can be used in the place of most store-bought baking mixes in various recipes, so if you have a recipe that calls for baking mix, you might want to try this recipe first instead of a store-bought version! Unlike most of my homemade mixes, which can be stored in your pantry, this mix should stay in the fridge, since we are adding butter to it before using it. You can also store it in the freezer if you don't plan on using it often or if you don't have the room to spare in your fridge.

You can use All-Purpose Gluten-Free Flour Mix (page 164) in this recipe. Just make sure to add some kind of binding agent as well, such as guar gum or xanthan gum.

―――――――― WHAT YOU NEED ――――――――

8 cups all-purpose flour (can be white or wheat)
⅓ cup baking powder
4 teaspoons salt
1 tablespoon sugar
1 cup vegetable oil, coconut oil,
or butter diced into small pieces

In a bowl, combine the flour, baking powder, sugar, and salt until well mixed. Add the oil or butter (we use coconut oil occasionally) and mix with a fork. Store in an airtight container in the refrigerator until ready to use.

Biscuits

―――――――― WHAT YOU NEED ――――――――

2½ cups All-Purpose Baking Mix
⅔ cup milk

Combine both ingredients in a bowl using a fork. Roll out the dough until it's at least ¾ inch thick. Cut out round biscuits with a biscuit cutter or with a glass cup that has been dipped in flour. Place the biscuits on a greased cookie sheet and bake at 350 degrees for 15 to 20 minutes or until the biscuits are slightly brown on top.

For dairy-free biscuits, use a nondairy milk such as almond or coconut milk.

You don't have to make plain biscuits if you don't want to! Here are some fun add-ins to try.

- ½ cup shredded cheddar cheese
- ½ cup shredded cheddar cheese and 2 tablespoons cooked, chopped bacon
- ¼ cup fruit preserves (only add ½ cup milk with this add-in)
- 1 teaspoon garlic salt and ½ cup shredded cheddar cheese
- 1 teaspoon minced onion and 1 tablespoon cream cheese

You could also add some honey butter to top off your biscuits. It's so good and easy to make! Simply whip 1 stick (½ cup) softened butter with 2 tablespoons honey. You can also add a pinch of ground cinnamon if you wish. For dairy-free honey butter, soften ½ cup coconut butter and whip with 2 tablespoons honey.

Chicken Pot Pie

——— WHAT YOU NEED ———

1 cup All-Purpose Baking Mix (page 171)

1 egg

1½ cups milk or cream

2 cups diced, cooked veggies (such as carrots, green beans, broccoli, peas, corn, etc.)

1 cup cooked, shredded chicken

¾ cup chicken stock or broth

1 teaspoon salt

In a bowl, mix together the baking mix, egg, and ½ cup milk. Set aside. In another large bowl, toss together the veggies, chicken, 1 cup milk, chicken stock, and salt. Pour the chicken mixture into a pie plate. Spread the baking mix mixture over the top. Bake at 400 degrees for 30 minutes or until the topping is crisp and brown.

For a dairy-free version, use a nondairy milk such as almond or coconut milk, or replace the 1 cup of milk (in the actual pie) with chicken broth.

Dumpling Soup

WHAT YOU NEED

2 cups All-Purpose Baking Mix (page 171)

⅔ cup milk

6 cups chicken broth

½ cup apple juice

2 cups chopped, cooked veggies (celery, carrots, peas, corn, etc.)

1 teaspoon salt

1 teaspoon minced onion

½ teaspoon garlic powder

1 cup cooked, shredded chicken

In a bowl, mix together the milk and baking mix until it forms a dough. Place all the remaining ingredients together in a large saucepan on medium heat. Once the soup is simmering, add the dough one tablespoon at a time. Cook the dumplings in the soup for about 20 minutes and serve warm.

For dairy-free dumplings, use a nondairy milk such as almond or coconut milk.

Money-Saving Tip: Take advantage of farmers' markets when searching for fresh food. Make sure to look at all the vendors before you make your choices. Go at the end of the day, when farmers are looking to sell off what they have left, and always ask if they have bulk pricing available.

rice side mix

· · ·

I'm definitely not a side dish maker. I can put together a yummy main dish, but I tend to serve it with just a bowl of fresh green beans or buttered corn or something else simple that I can pull out of my garden or from my home-canned jars of food. This rice mix opened up our side dish possibilities a bit and added some extra flavor. I've also used these mixes to create a yummy soup base (I just add the mix, some broth, cooked meat, and veggies and it's a meal!) or as a bed for a simple cooked chicken breast.

There are many possibilities with these recipes no matter how you use them and they are a great pantry staple to have on hand at all times!

WHAT YOU NEED

¾ cup uncooked rice
½ cup uncooked spaghetti or orzo
½ teaspoon garlic powder
½ teaspoon onion powder
1 teaspoon salt

Break the spaghetti into small pieces. You can use orzo if you are in a hurry or want to skip this step. Add all the ingredients together in a jar. (This recipe fits into a pint jar or a quart storage bag.)

Rice Side Dish

WHAT YOU NEED

1 recipe Rice Side Mix
2 tablespoons butter
2 cups chicken or vegetable broth or stock

Brown the butter in a skillet. Add the mix and chicken or vegetable broth. Cook (stirring frequently) until rice and pasta are cooked through.

To make a gluten-free version, use gluten-free pasta.

To make a dairy-free version, use coconut oil instead of butter.

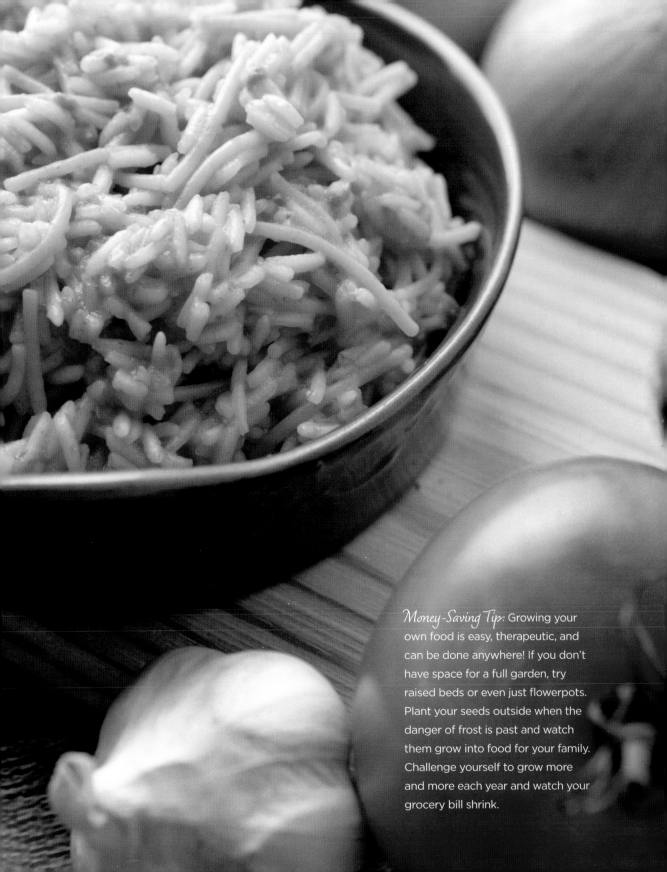

Money-Saving Tip: Growing your own food is easy, therapeutic, and can be done anywhere! If you don't have space for a full garden, try raised beds or even just flowerpots. Plant your seeds outside when the danger of frost is past and watch them grow into food for your family. Challenge yourself to grow more and more each year and watch your grocery bill shrink.

Herbed Garlic Rice Side Dish Mix

½ cup uncooked spaghetti

¾ cup uncooked rice

1 teaspoon minced garlic

½ teaspoon dried parsley

1 teaspoon salt

Create the mix and recipe using the same instructions as for the classic dish on page 174. You may also want to add a bit of chopped green onion just before serving.

Spanish Rice Side Dish Mix

WHAT YOU NEED

½ cup uncooked spaghetti

¾ cup uncooked rice

1 teaspoon salt

1 teaspoon minced onion

1 tablespoon dried tomato powder

½ teaspoon chili powder

Create the mix and recipe using the same instructions as for the classic dish on page 174. We like to serve this version with a bit of sour cream on top. If you cannot find dried tomato powder, substitute a cup of fresh diced tomatoes in place of 1 cup of chicken broth when cooking.

To make a gluten-free version, use gluten-free pasta.

To make a dairy-free version, use coconut oil instead of butter.

Note: You can make your own dried tomato powder to add to mixes if needed. Simply slice up fresh tomatoes into very thin pieces, place them in a food dehydrator, and dry for at least 10 hours at 150 degrees. If your oven goes to a low temp, you can try this in there as well on a baking sheet; just make sure to watch the tomatoes very carefully so they don't burn. Keep the dried tomatoes in an airtight container (or in the freezer) until ready to use. You can store them whole or grind them into a powder to take up less space.

faux bouillon

· · ·

You know those little cubes of something that claims to be chicken or beef or vegetable broth that they sell at the store? Yeah, you really shouldn't buy or consume those. Not only are you missing out on some great flavor from healthy homemade stock, you are usually adding a dose of MSG or other chemicals into your diet with them. While this recipe isn't exactly the same, it's good enough to replace it in many mix recipes. In recipes where you need a large amount of bouillon or broth, it would be better to use fresh homemade stock. You can find nutritional yeast flakes at most health food stores.

―――――― WHAT YOU NEED ――――――

1½ cups nutritional yeast flakes

2½ tablespoons salt

1½ tablespoons minced onion

1½ tablespoons dried parsley

1 teaspoon dried sage

1 teaspoon celery seed

1½ teaspoons garlic powder

1 teaspoon dried thyme

1 teaspoon dried marjoram

1 teaspoon dried rosemary

1 teaspoon paprika

½ teaspoon dried basil

Mix all the ingredients together until well blended. Store in a pint jar and use as needed.

chicken noodle soup mix

· · ·

There isn't anything better than a warm bowl of soup on a cold day or on a day when you aren't feeling your best. Chicken noodle soup (or chicken and rice soup if we replace the noodles with rice) is our older son's very favorite meal. I'm not sure where he puts it all, but when I make this dish for supper he can eat several bowls full in one sitting! The chicken noodle soup recipe is great because it can be made on the stovetop just half an hour before supper. The Chili Mix (page 179) can be placed right in the slow cooker for a meal you can put together in the morning and have ready by suppertime.

─────── WHAT YOU NEED ───────

1 cup uncooked egg noodles
2 tablespoons Faux Bouillon (page 177)
½ teaspoon pepper
¼ teaspoon dried thyme
⅛ teaspoon celery seeds
¼ teaspoon garlic powder
1 teaspoon salt

Mix all the ingredients together and store in a jar or storage bag.

Chicken Noodle Soup

─────── WHAT YOU NEED ───────

1 recipe Chicken Noodle Soup Mix
8 cups filtered water
2 carrots, diced
2 stalks celery, diced
1 small onion, diced
3 cups cooked, cubed chicken

Add all the ingredients to a large saucepan and simmer on the stove for 30 minutes or until vegetables and noodles are cooked through.

To make this soup gluten-free, use gluten-free pasta.

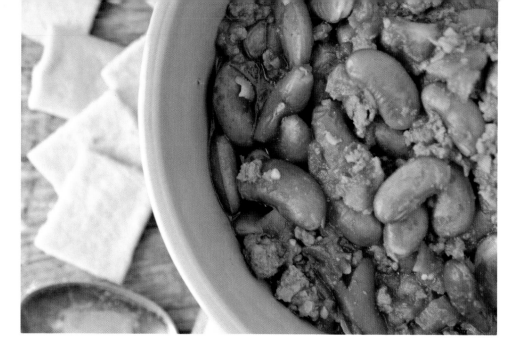

chili mix

· · ·

3 cups dried kidney beans   *1 teaspoon cumin*

2 tablespoons chili powder   *½ teaspoon oregano*

2 tablespoons minced onion   *¼ teaspoon cayenne pepper*

1 tablespoon garlic salt

Mix all the ingredients together in a bowl and place in a quart jar or a storage bag.

Chili

1 pound ground beef   *2 cups (16 ounces) diced tomatoes*

1 recipe Chili Mix   *Shredded cheddar cheese*

6 cups filtered water   *Sour cream*

Brown the ground beef and place in the slow cooker with the other ingredients. Cook on the high setting for 8 hours or until the beans are tender. Serve warm with a sprinkle of cheddar cheese and a dollop of sour cream.

onion soup mix

. . .

Onion Soup Mix is another all-purpose mix that is great for seasoning meats and veggies and making yummy dips! Just a few ingredients are all you need.

——————— WHAT YOU NEED ———————

¾ cup minced onion

⅓ cup Faux Bouillon (page 177)

4 teaspoons onion powder

¼ teaspoon sugar

¼ teaspoon celery seed

Mix all the ingredients together and store in a small jar. Use as needed.

cream of soup mix

. . .

You know all those cans of cream of whatever soup that you've been buying? After you make this recipe, you won't need those anymore . . . any of them! This is a general "cream of soup" mix that is a perfect replacement for cream of mushroom soup, cream of chicken soup, and more. Plus, instead of needing the space to store all of those cans, you can simply store this bulk mix in a large jar and take up much less space in your pantry.

──────────── WHAT YOU NEED ────────────

2 cups powdered milk or powdered coconut milk
2½ cups all-purpose flour or
All-Purpose Gluten-Free Flour Mix (page 164)
¼ cup Faux Bouillon (page 177)
2 tablespoons minced onion

Mix all of these ingredients together in a bowl and pour into a large jar or storage bag.

Cream of Soup

──────────── WHAT YOU NEED ────────────

½ cup Cream of Soup Mix
1¼ cups warm filtered water

Combine the mix and the water. Stir until the mixture thickens slightly. If you need it to be very thick for a recipe, simmer it for a bit over medium heat.

For Cream of Chicken Soup: Add bits of cooked chicken as well if desired.

For Cream of Mushroom Soup: Add ¼ cup diced mushrooms.

For Cream of Celery Soup: Add ¼ cup finely diced celery or 1 teaspoon celery seed.

For Cream of Potato Soup: Add ½ cup mashed potatoes.

Money-Saving Tip: A clean kitchen will save not only time but money. Try to clean out your refrigerator and pantry about once a month so you know exactly what you have on hand and can prevent yourself from buying excess and letting products expire.

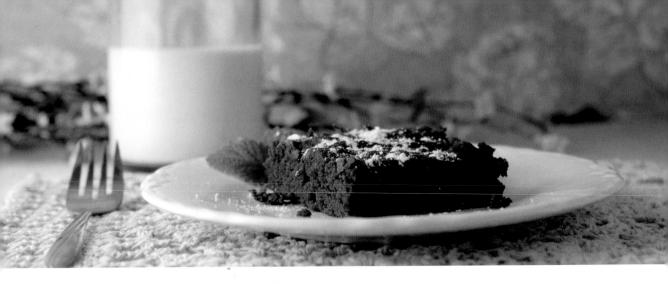

brownie mix

· · ·

Everyone needs a special treat once in a while, and who doesn't love a delicious brownie? We use this simple brownie mix for all kinds of different snacks and desserts and it's well worth having on your pantry shelf. This is my normally-I-wouldn't-have-time-to-make-dessert-but-the-brownie-mix-was-already-sitting-on-my-shelf recipe! And if just thinking about brownies hasn't convinced you to make this yet, take a peek at some of the following recipes that you can make using this delicious mix.

A boxed brownie mix can cost well over $3 for a regular version or over $5 for a gluten-free version. This homemade recipe costs less than $1 per mix and there are no questionable ingredients here. If you make one box of gluten-free brownie mix per week, you would save over $208 per year making the homemade version instead. Think of all the other things you could buy with an extra $200 a year instead of brownies!

─────── WHAT YOU NEED ───────

1⅓ cups all-purpose flour or
All-Purpose Gluten-Free Flour Mix (page 164)
1 cup sugar
⅓ cup unsweetened cocoa powder
½ teaspoon baking powder
½ teaspoon salt

Mix all the ingredients together until well blended. Store in a pint-size mason jar or a quart storage bag.

Brownies

WHAT YOU NEED

1 recipe Brownie Mix (page 182)
½ cup filtered water
½ cup vegetable oil
1 teaspoon vanilla extract

Mix together all the ingredients in a large bowl until they are well combined. Pour into a greased 8x8-inch baking dish and bake at 350 degrees for 20 minutes. Enjoy warm or topped with a scoop of ice cream for a special treat.

Brownie Bites

WHAT YOU NEED

1 recipe Brownie Mix (page 182)
½ cup filtered water
½ cup vegetable oil
1 teaspoon vanilla extract
½ cup mini chocolate chips

In a large bowl, mix together all the ingredients. You may need more chocolate chips in your recipe, depending on how "chocolate chippy" you want your brownie bites to be. Scoop the batter by teaspoonful into a greased mini muffin pan. Bake at 350 degrees for 15 to 20 minutes.

Other fun things you can add to your brownie bites instead of chocolate chips:

- ½ cup blueberries
- ½ cup dried cranberries
- ½ cup butterscotch chips
- 1 teaspoon mint extract (instead of vanilla)
- 2 tablespoons espresso powder or instant coffee
- ½ cup chopped nuts
- ½ cup peanut butter
- ⅓ cup raspberry jam

You can also add any of these into the regular brownie recipe as well!

Fudge Cookies

WHAT YOU NEED

8 ounces cream cheese
½ cup butter, softened or melted
½ recipe Brownie Mix (page 182)

In a bowl, mix the cream cheese and butter. Add the brownie mix and stir well. Drop by teaspoonful onto a greased cookie sheet and bake at 350 degrees for 10 to 15 minutes. Cookies may be slightly "doughy" in the middle but this will allow them to remain soft.

Brownie Whoopie Pies

WHAT YOU NEED

1 recipe Brownie Mix (page 182)
2 eggs
½ cup filtered water
¼ cup vegetable oil
1 cup butter, softened
3 to 4 cups confectioners' sugar

In a large bowl, combine the brownie mix, eggs, water, and oil. The mixture should be somewhat thin. Grease a bar pan or cookie sheet well and pour small amounts of batter in circles onto the pan (like you are making small pancakes). Bake at 400 degrees for 8 to 10 minutes.

In another bowl, mix together the softened butter with the powdered sugar. Using an electric hand mixer, whip the filling until light and fluffy. If the filling is too rich for you, replace ½ cup butter with ½ cup cream cheese.

Note: If you don't have any confectioners' sugar on hand, you can make your own! Mix 1 cup granulated sugar with 1 tablespoon cornstarch and blend together in a food processor until powdered. To replace the powdered sugar for this entire recipe you will need 3 to 4 cups of sugar and 3 to 4 tablespoons of cornstarch, but I recommend only blending 1 cup at a time.

Layered Cheesecake Brownies

———— WHAT YOU NEED ————

1 recipe Brownie Mix (page 182)

½ cup filtered water

½ cup vegetable oil

4 ounces cream cheese, softened

½ teaspoon vanilla extract

1 egg

In a bowl, mix together the brownie mix, water, and oil. Set aside. In another bowl, mix together the softened cream cheese, vanilla, and egg.

Spread two-thirds of the brownie batter in the bottom of a greased 8x8-inch baking dish. Drop the cheesecake batter by tablespoonful onto the top of the brownie batter. Pour the rest of the brownie batter over the cheesecake batter. Run a knife through the combined batters to create a swirl effect.

Bake at 350 degrees for 35 to 40 minutes. Cool before enjoying.

Brownie Batter Fudge

———— WHAT YOU NEED ————

1 cup Brownie Mix (page 182)

1 cup confectioners' sugar

½ cup butter, diced into small pieces

¼ cup milk

Grease an 8x8-inch baking dish well. Place all the ingredients in a medium bowl and microwave for 2 minutes. Remove from the microwave and stir quickly until all the ingredients are combined. Pour into the prepared pan and cool for at least 2 hours or until set. Cut into small squares and serve.

For a dairy-free version of this fudge, use coconut oil instead of the butter and a nondairy milk for the milk.

For a chocolate mint flavor, add a few drops of mint extract!

Money-Saving Tip: Keep a firm grocery budget each month and make sure it's in cash. Plan out your grocery list and meals accordingly, and once the money is gone, it's gone, so learn to make the most of that budget.

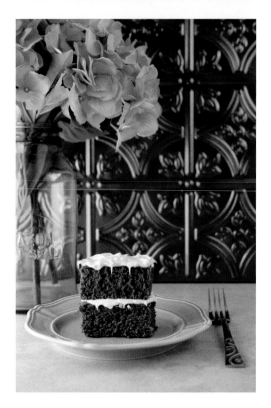

cake mix

. . .

Today, boxed cake mix at the store usually costs between $2 and $3 per box. This recipe costs only around $0.75 per cake mix, and believe me when I say that these homemade cakes taste so much fresher than anything from a box.

In the Little House on the Prairie books, we read about how, right before her wedding, Laura was beating egg whites by hand for her wedding cake until they were stiff. (Can you imagine?!) I can promise you that these cake recipes aren't nearly as strenuous but will produce the same amazing results.

Cake mixes are great because they aren't just good for cakes but for a host of desserts. We aren't big dessert eaters, but I love having some of this mix on hand for when a craving arises or a guest drops in.

Here are two basic cake or dessert mixes, yellow and chocolate. I'll share those with you first and then share a few of our favorite recipes to make with them!

Yellow Cake Mix

1½ cups all-purpose flour or
All-Purpose Gluten-Free Flour Mix
(page 164)

3 teaspoons baking powder
¼ teaspoon salt
¾ cup sugar

Combine all the ingredients and store in a jar or storage bag.

Yellow Cake

1 recipe Yellow Cake Mix
¼ cup butter, softened
1 teaspoon vanilla extract

3 eggs
½ cup milk

Cream the dry mix with the butter, vanilla, and eggs. Add the milk slowly and stir well. Pour into a greased 9x13-inch baking pan and bake at 375 degrees for 25 to 30 minutes or until a toothpick poked into the center of the cake comes out clean.

For a dairy-free version, use a nondairy milk and ¼ cup of coconut oil or coconut butter instead of regular butter.

See below for fun variations.

Simple Variations for Yellow Cake

For a denser, slightly spongy cake, use orange juice in place of the milk.
Add ½ cup chopped nuts into the batter.
Add ½ cup mini chocolate chips into the batter.
Bake in a muffin pan for cupcakes.
Swirl ½ cup raspberry preserves into the batter.
For a spice cake, add 1 teaspoon cinnamon, ¼ teaspoon ground cloves, and ¼ teaspoon allspice to the batter.
Pineapple Upside-Down Cake: Melt ½ cup butter with ½ cup brown sugar and pour the mixture in the bottom of the pan first. Top with sliced pineapple, and follow with the batter. Invert cake before serving.
Add ½ cup chopped dried apricots to the batter.

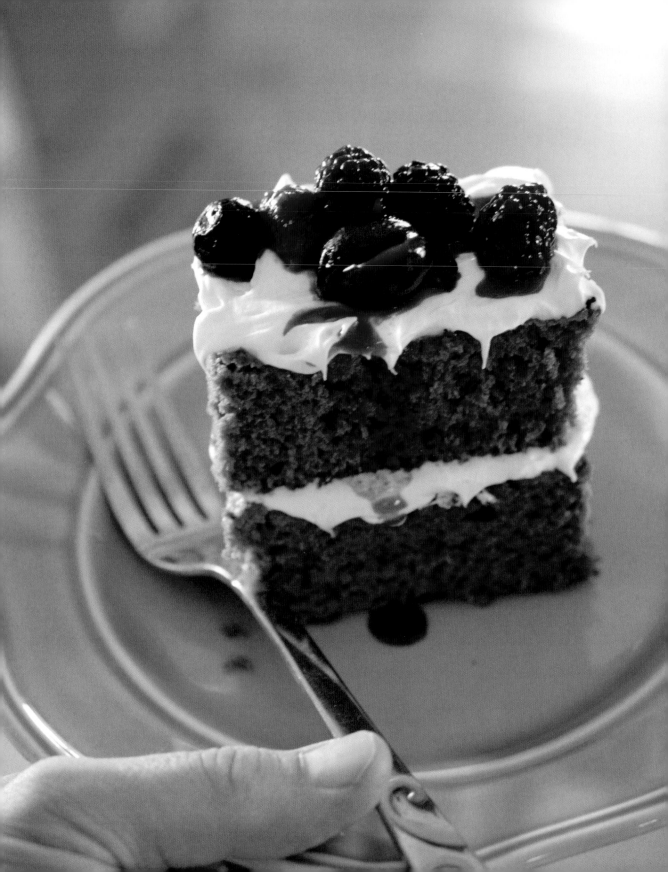

Chocolate Cake Mix

WHAT YOU NEED

1½ cups sugar

2 cups all-purpose flour or
All-Purpose Gluten-Free
Flour Mix (page 164)

2 teaspoons baking powder

½ teaspoon salt

⅓ cup unsweetened cocoa powder

Combine all the ingredients and store in a jar or storage bag.

Chocolate Cake

WHAT YOU NEED

1 recipe Chocolate Cake Mix

½ cup melted butter or oil

1 teaspoon vanilla extract

2 eggs

1 cup milk

Cream the dry cake mix with the melted butter or oil, vanilla, and eggs. Add the milk slowly and stir well. Pour into a greased 9x13-inch baking pan and bake at 350 degrees for 30 minutes or until a toothpick poked into the center of the cake comes out clean.

For a dairy-free version of this cake, use a nondairy milk and ½ cup coconut oil or coconut butter instead of regular butter.

See below for fun variations.

Simple Variations for Chocolate Cake

For a denser cake, use ½ cup less flour in the mix and add ½ cup mashed potatoes to the batter.

Add 1 cup chopped pecans into the batter.

Use ½ cup sour cream and ½ cup milk instead of 1 cup milk.

For a spice cake, add 1 teaspoon cinnamon, ¼ teaspoon ground cloves, and ¼ teaspoon allspice to the batter.

Swirl raspberry or strawberry preserves into the batter before baking or simply add ½ cup of preserves directly into the batter while mixing.

Add ½ cup chocolate chips into the batter for double chocolate.

Add ½ cup shredded coconut to the batter.

Chocolate Mint Cake: Add 1 teaspoon mint extract instead of vanilla extract.

Replace one of the eggs with a mashed banana.

Add 1 teaspoon instant coffee or espresso powder to the batter.

There are so many fun things you can do with a basic cake mix! Here are some other dessert recipes that you can try with the mixes.

Dump Cake

─────── WHAT YOU NEED ───────

4 cups frozen or fresh blueberries
½ cup sugar
1 recipe Yellow Cake Mix (page 187)
¾ cup butter, melted
Whipped cream

In a small bowl, mix together the blueberries and sugar, and pour into a 9x13-inch baking dish. Sprinkle the dry cake mix over the top of the blueberries to form an even layer. Pour the melted butter over the top of the cake mix. Bake at 350 degrees for 50 minutes to 1 hour. The top should be golden brown when it's ready. Serve with a bit of fresh whipped cream.

For a dairy-free version, replace the butter with coconut oil or coconut butter.

Soft and Creamy Cookies

─────── WHAT YOU NEED ───────

1 recipe Chocolate Cake Mix (page 189)
8 ounces cream cheese, softened
1 egg
½ teaspoon vanilla extract

In a large bowl, mix together all the ingredients. Drop onto a well-greased cookie sheet by teaspoonful and bake at 350 degrees for 12 to 15 minutes. Cookies will be soft when removed from the oven.

Dessert Waffles

WHAT YOU NEED

1 recipe Chocolate Cake Mix (page 189)

3 eggs

1⅓ cups filtered water

⅓ cup vegetable oil

Fresh berries

Whipped cream

In a large bowl, mix all the ingredients together. Pour the batter onto a hot waffle iron (following the instructions that came with your waffle iron) and cook until done. Top with fresh berries and whipped cream.

Cinnamon Rolls

WHAT YOU NEED

2½ cups warm filtered water

4 teaspoons yeast

Pinch of sugar

1 recipe Yellow Cake Mix (page 187)

4½ cups all-purpose flour or

All-Purpose Gluten-Free Flour Mix (page 164)

½ cup butter, softened

½ cup brown sugar

2 teaspoons cinnamon

In a bowl, mix together the water and yeast with a pinch of sugar. Set aside until the yeast is foamy. In a large bowl, combine the cake mix and yeast mixture. Add the flour 1 cup at a time, stirring the dough and kneading between each addition until all the flour is added. Cover the dough with a clean towel and let it rise in a warm place for about an hour.

Punch down the dough and knead. Roll out the dough (on a floured surface) to form a rectangle no thicker than ¼ inch. Spread the softened butter over the dough and sprinkle with the brown sugar and cinnamon. Roll up the entire rectangle into a log and use a bread knife or sharp knife to cut into 1-inch-wide rolls. Place the rolls in a greased 9x13-inch baking pan and top with a bit of melted butter. Let the rolls rise again (covered with a clean towel) in a warm area for 30 minutes. Place the rolls in the oven at 375 degrees for 20 minutes or until the rolls are golden brown. You can top with additional melted butter or a simple glaze made with 1 cup confectioners' sugar and 3 tablespoons milk.

For a dairy-free version of these rolls, replace the butter in the recipe with coconut butter. You can skip the softened butter inside the rolls completely (or use a bit of coconut oil instead) and just sprinkle on cinnamon and sugar.

Honey Bun Cake

WHAT YOU NEED

1 recipe Yellow Cake Mix (page 187)
1 cup yogurt
4 eggs
¾ cup vegetable oil or melted butter
2 teaspoons cinnamon
1 cup brown sugar

In a large bowl, combine the cake mix, yogurt, eggs, and oil. In another small bowl, mix together the cinnamon and brown sugar. Spread ½ of the cake mix batter in the bottom of a greased 9x13-inch cake pan. Sprinkle the brown sugar mixture over the batter and top with the remaining batter. Cover the brown sugar evenly. Bake at 350 degrees for 40 minutes or until a toothpick poked in the middle of the cake comes out clean. For extra sweetness, top with a simple glaze made with 1 cup confectioners' sugar and 3 tablespoons milk.

For a dairy-free version, use 1 cup of full-fat (canned) coconut milk instead of yogurt.

Money-Saving Tip: If you use a lot of eggs and your city allows backyard chickens, you should give it a try! Hens are very quiet and just need good shelter, clean water, and plenty of bugs and food to eat and a bit of room to roam. The average hen produces an egg each day and a rooster isn't necessary for good egg production.

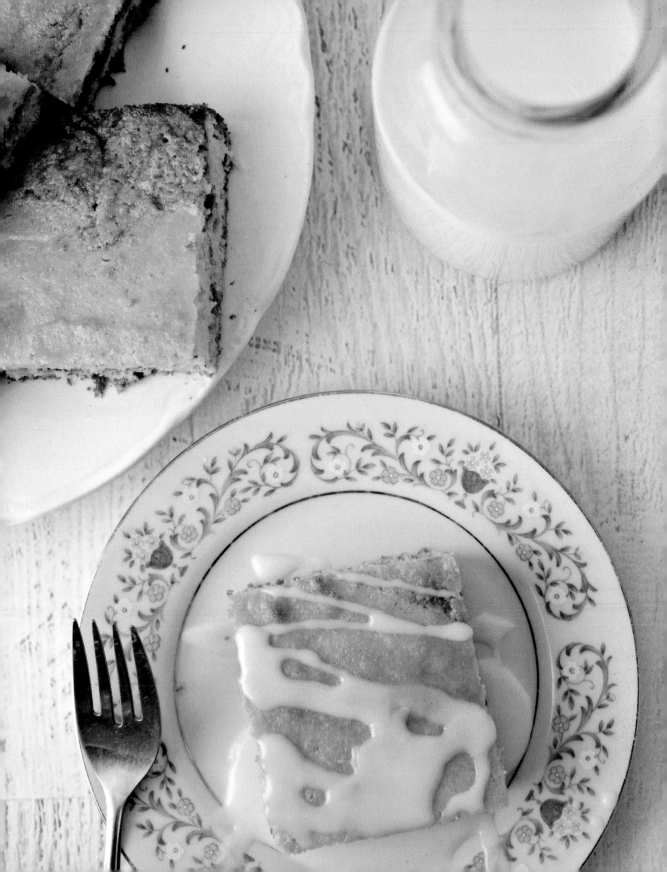

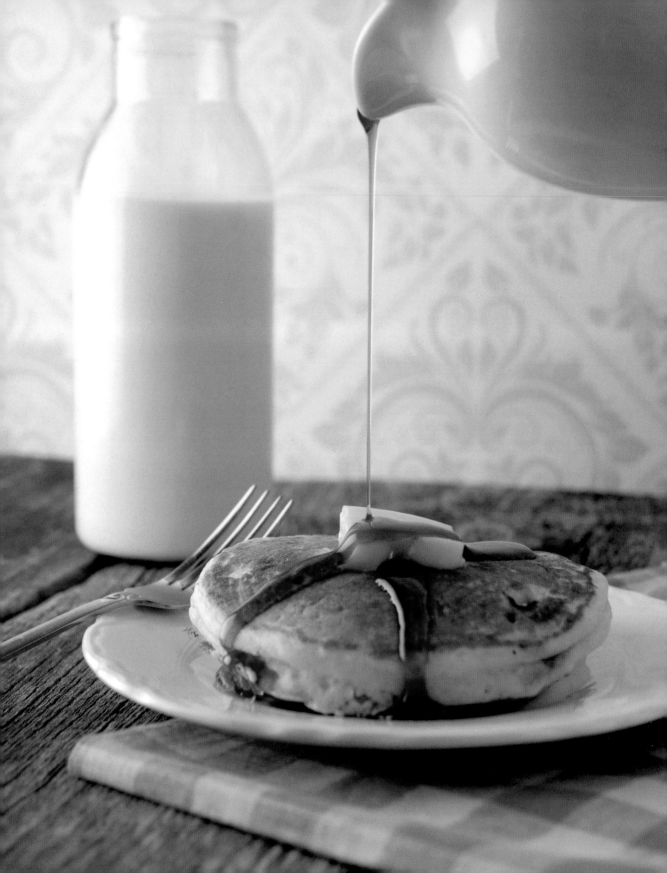

pancake and waffle mix

· · ·

When I was little, I spent a great deal of time with both sets of grandparents. I used to spend the night with my mother's parents fairly often. Since I'd been taught to cook at a very early age, one of my favorite things to do when I spent the night was to make them breakfast. I'd sneak out of bed in the morning and into the kitchen. I'd then proceed to be as quiet as I could while I prepared fruit, eggs, toast, and other things to make a breakfast feast. I'd set the table as fancy as I could, and then Granny and Grandpa would always appear at just the right time to enjoy their breakfast.

Now that I have a family of my own, I've realized my routine is somewhat similar. I head to the kitchen in the morning, and after my morning chores, I prepare breakfast for my little family so it's ready by the time they get up.

Keeping a large jar of this mix on hand at all times ensures that you can have quick breakfasts, and suppers too! This delicious mix has been my saving grace on many nights when five o'clock came around and I still didn't know what I was serving for supper. For breakfast we love to pair pancakes with fruits or fruit butters that we preserve in the fall, and for supper we serve the pancakes with butter and maple syrup and a side of homemade hash browns, eggs, and homemade sausage. Yum!

WHAT YOU NEED

4 cups all-purpose flour or
All-Purpose Gluten-Free Flour Mix (page 164)
2 teaspoons salt
¼ cup sugar
1 tablespoon and 1 teaspoon baking powder

Mix all the ingredients together well. Store in a quart jar or storage bag in the pantry until ready to use.

Basic Pa: /Waffles

———————— WHA   ¯ED ————————

1½ cups Panc∂.   ɔage 195)

1

3 tablespoons ɒutter, melted

½ cup milk

Whisk all the ingredients together until just blended; some lumps are okay. Heat a frying pan or griddle and pour small amounts of batter (we use a ¼-cup measure to pour out batter). If you aren't using a nonstick pan, melt a bit of butter in your frying pan or griddle before pouring the batter in. Cook the pancake until it begins to bubble and then flip and cook the other side. Fry until browned on both sides. You can also use this batter in a waffle iron; follow the directions of your individual model.

For dairy-free pancakes, use a milk replacement such as coconut or almond milk and replace the butter with coconut butter.

See below for some fun pancake add-ins.

Pancake Add-in Ideas

¼ cup mini chocolate chips
1 diced apple
1 diced banana
½ cup blueberries
¼ cup peanut butter
2 tablespoons lemon juice and 2 teaspoons poppy seeds
½ cup crumbled bacon
½ cup coconut milk (instead of regular milk) and ¼ cup shredded coconut
1 mashed banana and ½ cup diced strawberries
½ cup pureed pumpkin and 1 teaspoon pumpkin pie spice
¼ cup shredded zucchini
½ cup shredded cheddar cheese
½ cup diced peaches
½ cup yogurt (instead of milk)

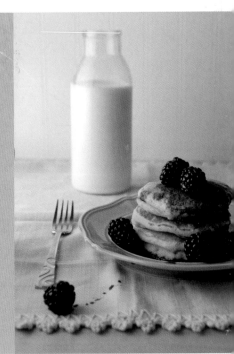

Making pancakes isn't the only thing you can do with pancake mix. It's also a great all-purpose mix, thanks to its basic ingredients! Here are a few other delicious recipes to try:

Fried Chicken

————— WHAT YOU NEED —————

Oil for frying
1 cup Pancake Mix (page 195)
¼ to ⅓ cup milk
2 cups cubed, uncooked chicken breast

In a medium saucepan on low to medium heat, start heating up the oil. In a bowl, combine the pancake mix and the milk. You want this mixture to be thicker than regular pancake mix but thinner than dough. Cube the chicken into pieces no larger than ½ inch thick. Dip the pieces of chicken in the batter and place into the hot oil (cover the oil with a lid while frying to help prevent splattering). Cook the chicken (you can cook several pieces at one time, but don't overcrowd the pan) for 2 minutes before turning and then for at least another 2 minutes, or until the inside of a cut-open piece of chicken is no longer pink and has reached at least 165 degrees when measured with a meat thermometer. Continue until all the chicken is cooked.

For a dairy-free version, use a nondairy milk such as coconut or almond milk.

Coffee Cake

WHAT YOU NEED

1 cup Pancake Mix (page 195)
¼ cup sugar
1 egg
⅓ cup milk
¼ cup butter, softened

Crumble Topping

WHAT YOU NEED

2 tablespoons butter, softened
1 tablespoon flour
2 tablespoons uncooked old-fashioned oats
¼ cup brown sugar

Mix the ingredients for the coffee cake together in a medium bowl. In a small bowl, combine the ingredients for the crumble topping. Pour the batter into a greased 8x8-inch baking dish. Crumble the topping over the batter. Bake the cake at 350 degrees for 20 minutes or until a toothpick inserted in the center of the cake comes out clean.

For a dairy-free version, use a nondairy milk such as coconut or almond milk and use coconut butter or coconut oil in place of the butter.

Oven Apple Pancake

WHAT YOU NEED

¾ cup brown sugar, divided   1½ cups Pancake Mix (page 195)
⅓ cup butter   2 eggs
½ cup maple syrup   1 cup milk
2 medium apples, diced

In a saucepan, combine ½ cup brown sugar, the butter, the maple syrup, and the apples. Simmer together for about 1 minute, until the sugar, butter, and syrup have combined thoroughly and liquefied. Pour into a greased 9x13-inch baking dish.

Combine the pancake mix, eggs, remaining ¼ cup brown sugar, and milk in a bowl. Pour the batter over the apple mixture in the baking dish. Bake at 350 degrees for 30 to 35 minutes. Cool slightly and cut into pieces and invert before serving. Can be topped with additional maple syrup and melted butter if desired.

For a dairy-free version, use a nondairy milk such as coconut or almond milk and use coconut butter or coconut oil in place of the butter.

Money-Saving Tip: In Laura Ingalls Wilder's books, sausage was made from scraps left over from butchering a pig. You can make it much more easily with ground pork, beef, chicken, or turkey. Combine 3 pounds of ground beef, pork, chicken, or turkey (or a mixture of several different meats). Add 3 teaspoons of salt and any of your favorite spices (such as thyme, sage, fennel, etc.). Let the mixture sit overnight in the fridge, then fry up and use as needed in your favorite breakfasts! Store any uncooked sausage in the freezer until ready to use.

muffin mix

. . .

Muffins are another fun item to have on hand. They can be used for snacks, breakfasts, side dishes, or even desserts, depending on what you fill them with!

This simple all-purpose mix can be made into endless varieties of muffins. First create the bulk mix and then check out all the add-in ideas to create unique and delicious muffins.

Usually, when we make muffins from this mix, I make a double batch, since I already have the oven on. We freeze the muffins from the second batch and my family then has fresh muffins that they can pull out of the freezer to enjoy when the first batch is gone. It saves me time and I'm not tempted to go to the store and pick up nonhomemade muffins, which saves us money!

———————— WHAT YOU NEED ————————

6 cups all-purpose flour or All-Purpose
Gluten-Free Flour Mix (page 164)
3 tablespoons baking powder
1½ teaspoons salt
½ cup sugar

Mix all the ingredients together well and store in a large jar (half-gallon jars work great) or a gallon storage bag.

Basic Muffins

———————— WHAT YOU NEED ————————

2¼ cups Muffin Mix
2 eggs
1 cup milk
¼ cup butter, softened
Add-ins (see page 201)

Mix together all the ingredients until just blended (do not overmix) and scoop into a muffin pan that has been greased or lined. Bake at 400 degrees for 15 minutes.

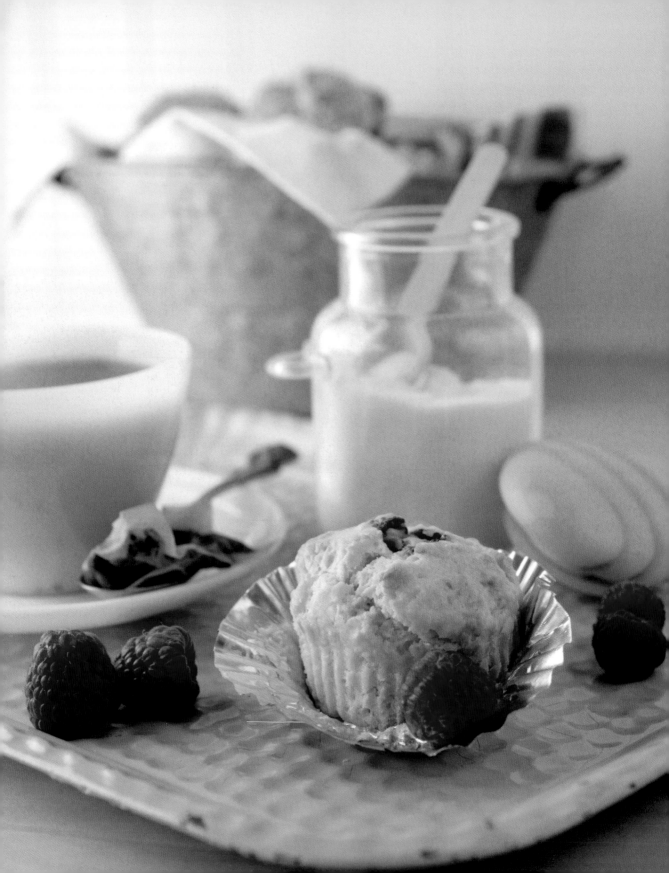

For dairy-free muffins, use a nondairy milk such as coconut or almond milk, and use coconut butter or coconut oil in place of the butter. See below for fun add-in ideas.

Money-Saving Tip: Make breads and meals ahead of time and freeze for the busy times. Muffins and quick breads are great items to bake and place in the freezer for when you need a quick and healthy snack. Freezing food will prevent impulse purchases when you are tired and don't feel like baking!

Muffin Add-in Ideas

BACON MUFFINS: ¼ cup crumbled, cooked bacon

BANANA MUFFINS: 1 mashed banana

BERRY MUFFINS: ½ cup blueberries, raspberries, or strawberries

CARROT MUFFINS: ½ cup shredded carrots, ½ teaspoon cinnamon, and ¼ teaspoon nutmeg

CHOCOLATE CHIP MUFFINS: ½ cup mini chocolate chips

CINNAMON RAISIN MUFFINS: ¼ cup raisins and 1 teaspoon cinnamon

PEACHES AND CREAM MUFFINS: ½ cup diced peaches and replace ½ cup milk with sour cream

STRAWBERRY RHUBARB MUFFINS: ½ cup diced strawberries, ¼ cup diced rhubarb, and additional ¼ cup sugar

ZUCCHINI MUFFINS: 1 cup shredded zucchini and ½ teaspoon cinnamon

baked oatmeal mix

. . .

I love having breakfast ready to go in the morning for everyone. It's one less thing that I'll have to worry about and the best way to start off the day. Baked oatmeal is a delicious, hearty breakfast that can be prepared the night before and tossed right in the oven in the morning, fresh and warm. This is a great breakfast or brunch to have ready if you are having company and you don't want to spend a lot of time in the morning getting things prepared. There are many fun variations and additions you can put in baked oatmeal to make it tasty and it's a very budget-friendly meal.

This mix makes baked oatmeal even easier to toss together and have when you need it!

———————— WHAT YOU NEED ————————

3 cups uncooked old-fashioned oats

1 teaspoon baking powder

½ teaspoon salt

2 tablespoons brown sugar

½ teaspoon cinnamon

¾ cup sugar

Mix all the ingredients together in a bowl and place in a quart jar or a storage bag.

Baked Oatmeal

———————— WHAT YOU NEED ————————

1 recipe Baked Oatmeal Mix

½ cup applesauce

2 eggs

1 cup milk

Combine all the ingredients in a bowl and stir thoroughly to mix. Pour into a greased 8x8-inch baking dish and place in the fridge overnight. In the morning, take out the dish and bake in the oven at 350 degrees for 35 minutes.

For a dairy-free version, use a nondairy milk such as coconut or almond milk.

There are so many things you could add to the batter to change up the recipe a bit!

- ½ cup shredded coconut
- ½ cup diced apples
- ½ cup diced peaches
- ½ cup diced cherries
- ½ cup whole blueberries
- ½ cup raisins
- ½ cup chopped strawberries
- ½ cup mini chocolate chips

For any of the fruits listed, you can use fresh or frozen fruit. Of course, if you have some home-canned fruits, you can use those as well!

Money-Saving Tip: Look for brown bananas or overly ripe produce at your grocery store and then find the produce manager, who will often give a great discount on riper items just to be able to sell them instead of having to throw them out. Ripe produce works great in smoothies, quick breads, and oatmeal and can be frozen to save until needed.

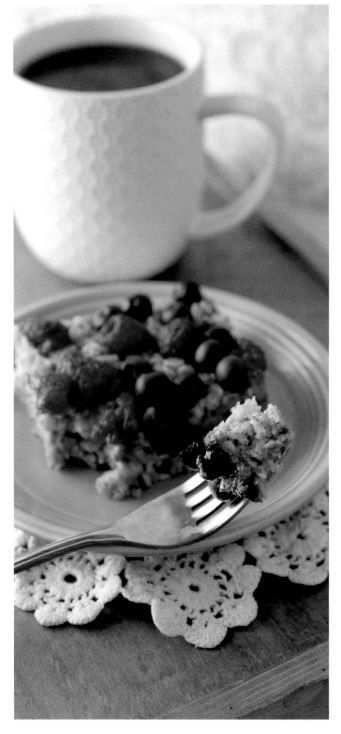

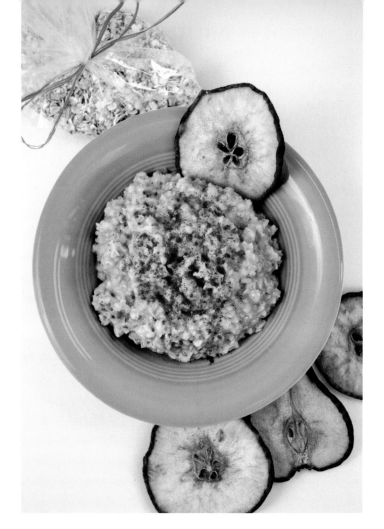

instant oatmeal packets

· · ·

I enjoy having oatmeal for breakfast year-round. There are so many different variations, it's easy to make, and it keeps my grocery budget lean and happy. At over $3
per box (of six or eight packages) for the store-bought varieties, you get breakfasts for
about a week, whereas if you spend that same amount of money on bulk oats, you can
stretch it out for months. When purchased in bulk, you can get oats for around $0.50
per pound, making it only pennies per serving.

But if you are still looking for that quick meal on the go that the instant oatmeal
packets make so convenient, you don't have to miss out by buying oats in bulk! They
are easy to make, and even easier to customize with your favorite flavors and varieties.

½ cup quick-cooking oats
2 teaspoons powdered milk or powdered coconut milk
1 tablespoon brown sugar

In a small bowl, mix all the ingredients until well combined. Place in a snack-size bag for a quick grab-and-go meal or snack. Add dried fruit and other ingredients to flavor as desired.

When you are ready to prepare your hot oatmeal, simply pour the packet into a bowl, add ¾ cup hot filtered water, stir, and enjoy.

If you don't need to separate your instant oatmeal into small grab-and-go packets, you can also mix it up in bulk and save yourself time, money, and the cost of the bags.

Bulk Instant Oatmeal

WHAT YOU NEED

5 cups quick-cooking oats
½ cup powdered milk or powdered coconut milk
⅔ cup brown sugar

Mix all the ingredients together in a large bowl and pour into a container to store. When you are ready to enjoy a bowl of oatmeal, mix ½ cup oatmeal mix with ¾ cup hot filtered water.

There are many fun additions you can add to either the bulk mix or the individual packets. Here are some ideas to get you started!

- Any dried fruit
- Cinnamon and raisins
- Powdered peanut butter
- Dried banana and chopped walnuts
- Dried apple and cinnamon
- White chocolate chips and dried cranberries
- Chocolate chips
- Hot Chocolate Mix (page 216), using hot milk instead of water
- Graham crackers

Money-Saving Tip: Shop along the perimeter of the grocery store. Almost all the middle aisles are filled with boxed and canned processed products that you (and your wallet) don't need!

pudding mix

· · ·

Pudding Mix is a fun thing to have around to make delicious pudding or to add to various recipes that call for pudding mix. While this isn't an "instant" pudding (you do have a bit of cooking time), it still saves time to have it premixed, and the cost savings of homemade mix versus store-bought mix can be significant! Not to mention that you can actually pronounce all the ingredients in this pudding recipe . . .

Each of these mix recipes will make several batches (one batch will serve 4 to 6 people) of fresh pudding.

Chocolate Pudding Mix

——— WHAT YOU NEED ———

1¼ cups sugar

1 cup cornstarch

1 cup powdered milk or powdered coconut milk

¼ cup unsweetened cocoa powder

¼ teaspoon salt

Mix all the ingredients thoroughly and store in a jar or a storage bag.

Chocolate Pudding

——— WHAT YOU NEED ———

½ cup Chocolate Pudding Mix

2 cups milk

½ teaspoon vanilla extract

In a saucepan over medium heat, whisk the pudding mix and the milk together. Stir and simmer until thickened. Remove from the heat and mix in the vanilla extract. Pour into a bowl or mugs and let it cool in the fridge before serving.

For a dairy-free version, use a nondairy milk such as coconut or almond milk.

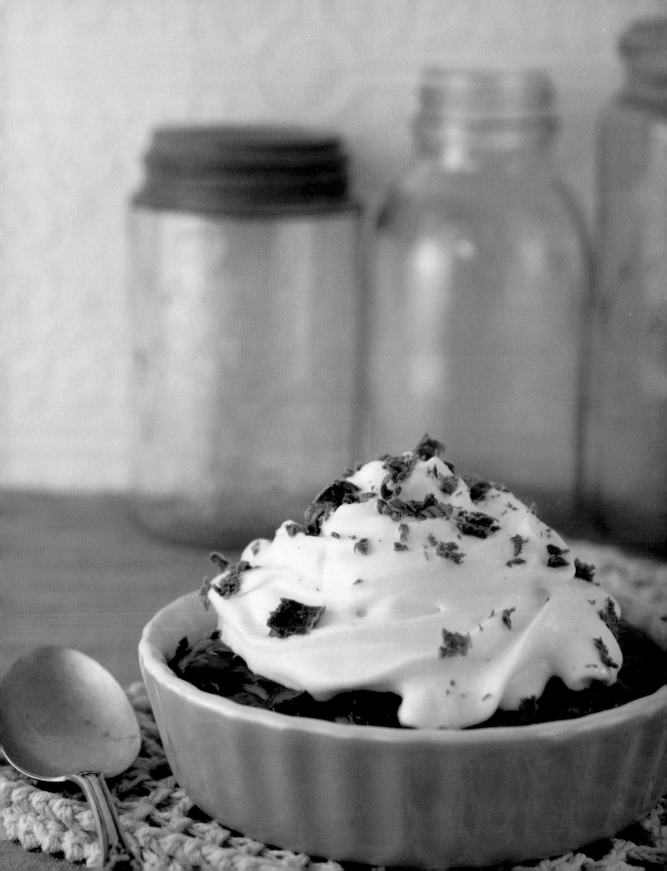

Pudding Variations

BANANA PUDDING: Add 3 sliced bananas into vanilla pudding.

CHEESECAKE PUDDING: Whip 4 ounces softened cream cheese into cooled chocolate or vanilla pudding until smooth.

CHOCOLATE CHIP PUDDING: Stir ½ cup mini chocolate chips into cooled vanilla or chocolate pudding before serving.

COCONUT PUDDING: Add coconut milk instead of regular milk when cooking the pudding and add ½ cup shredded coconut.

FUDGE PUDDING: Make the vanilla pudding recipe and add ½ cup chocolate chips while cooking. Cook until chips are melted.

Vanilla Pudding Mix

WHAT YOU NEED

1¼ cups sugar

1 cup cornstarch

1 cup powdered milk or powdered coconut milk

¼ teaspoon salt

Mix all the ingredients thoroughly and store in a jar or storage bag.

Vanilla Pudding

WHAT YOU NEED

½ cup Vanilla Pudding Mix

2 cups milk

1 teaspoon vanilla extract

In a saucepan over medium heat, whisk the pudding mix and the milk together. Stir and simmer until thickened. Remove from the heat and mix in the vanilla extract. Pour into a bowl or mugs and let it cool in the fridge before serving.

For a dairy-free version, use a nondairy milk such as coconut or almond milk.

Money-Saving Tip: Being able to make many variations from basic recipes is a huge money saver. Instead of trying to make the recipe with ingredients you have to buy, you can simply make the basic recipe and add ingredients that you have on hand to make it special.

chocolate chip cookie mix

. . .

This is one of our family's favorites, and I have been making this recipe since I was a young girl. I remember making these delicious cookies after school for a special snack for my entire family and I always would make them HUGE using the muffin scoop instead of the cookie scoop. If you are going to go for a cookie, you might as well make it worthwhile, right?

After I got married I turned this recipe into an easy mix that we could keep in our pantry for when we wanted a sweet treat. I hope it will become a family favorite at your home as well!

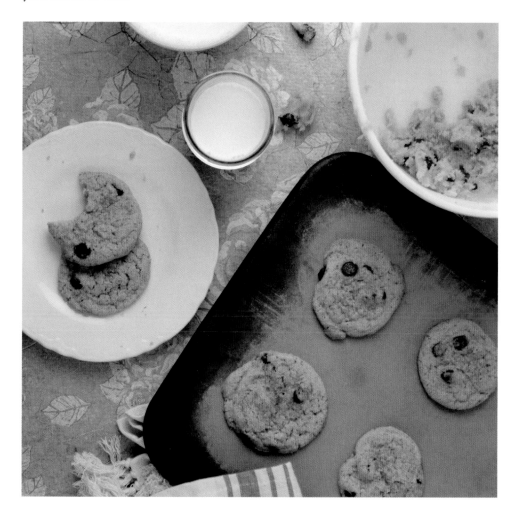

Chocolate Chip Cookie Mix

——————————— WHAT YOU NEED ———————————

¾ cup granulated sugar   1 teaspoon baking soda

¾ cup brown sugar   1 teaspoon salt

2¼ cups all-purpose flour or   2 cups chocolate chips

All-Purpose Gluten-Free

Flour Mix (page 164)

Mix together all the ingredients until well blended. Store in a jar or storage bag until ready to make cookies.

Chocolate Chip Cookies

——————————— WHAT YOU NEED ———————————

1 recipe Chocolate Chip Cookie Mix   1 cup butter, softened

2 eggs   1½ teaspoons vanilla extract

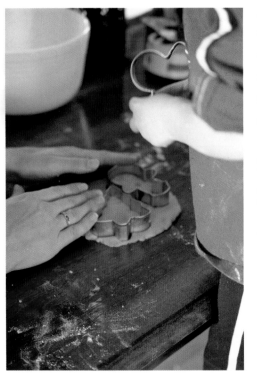

Mix all the ingredients together thoroughly. Drop the dough by teaspoonful (or tablespoonful!) onto a greased cookie sheet. Bake at 350 degrees for 12 minutes or until the tops of the cookies are slightly browned. These cookies should remain slightly soft.

For a dairy-free cookie, use coconut butter in place of the regular butter.

Money-Saving Tip: Chocolate chips can be quite expensive. Stock up on them during the holiday season while they are on sale and freeze what you don't need to use right away. Chocolate chips will last for months in the freezer!

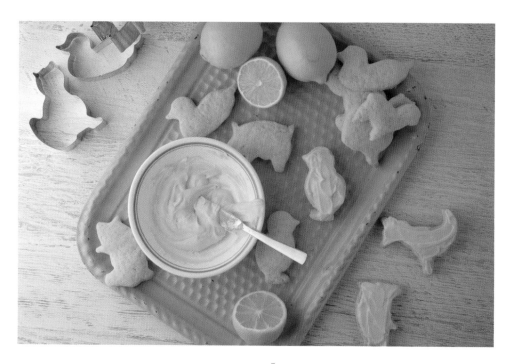

sugar cookie mix

. . .

During our first year at our little farm, I found a miniature donkey for sale and decided that I needed to bring him home. Few people know that donkeys are great protection for your other animals, so they are great to have around if you keep any kind of livestock . . . kind of like a big puppy! My little donkey's name is Charlie and he is nothing but a fluffy, lovable teddy bear. He will follow you around the pasture and nibble on your shirt looking for treats and a little scratching under his neck. Charlie has reminded me that everyone in this life deserves a cookie from time to time as a little treat for being a part of the family. Charlie's cookies are made from molasses, carrots, oats, and other yummy things that he likes. But one of our (our, as in, the humans at our farm!) favorite cookies are these delicious, soft sugar cookies. I made this recipe while I was growing up and I will always have fond memories of decorating these cookies with my family. This cookie mix is also a versatile one and can be used for quite a few different dessert recipes.

Like my chocolate chip cookies, I used to make these as big as possible by looking for the largest cookie cutter in the drawer!

Sugar Cookie Mix

1 cup sugar   *½ teaspoon salt*

2½ cups all-purpose flour   *½ teaspoon baking soda*

Mix all the ingredients until combined thoroughly and store in a jar or storage bag.

Sugar Cookies

1 recipe Sugar Cookie Mix   *½ teaspoon vanilla extract*

1 egg   *½ cup sour cream*

½ cup butter, softened

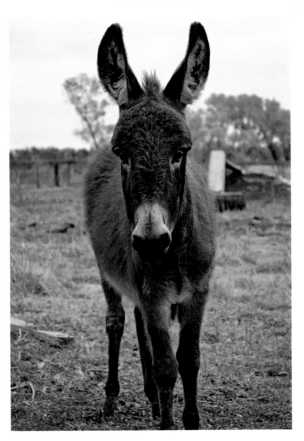

Mix all the ingredients together in a large bowl until well blended. Roll out the dough on a floured surface and cut into various shapes with cookie cutters. Place on a greased cookie sheet and bake at 350 degrees for 10 to 12 minutes or until the cookies begin to turn brown on the bottom. Decorate with frosting if desired or enjoy plain.

We've discovered that the following recipe works much better for dairy-free and gluten-free sugar cookies. These are just as tasty as the recipe above!

Dairy-Free, Gluten-Free Sugar Cookie Mix

─────────────── WHAT YOU NEED ───────────────

1½ cups sugar
3 cups All-Purpose Gluten-Free Flour Mix (page 164)
½ teaspoon salt
1 teaspoon baking powder

Mix all the ingredients until combined thoroughly and store in a jar or storage bag.

Dairy-Free, Gluten-Free Sugar Cookies

─────────────── WHAT YOU NEED ───────────────

1 recipe Dairy-Free, Gluten-Free Sugar Cookie Mix
1 cup coconut butter, softened
2 teaspoons vanilla extract
½ to ¾ cup coconut milk (full-fat, canned)

Mix all the ingredients together in a large bowl until well blended. Roll out the dough on a floured surface and cut into various shapes with cookie cutters. Place on a greased cookie sheet and bake at 350 degrees for 15 to 20 minutes or until cookies begin to turn brown on the bottom.

Here are some other fun recipes to try with your sugar cookie mix. If using the dairy-free, gluten-free version of the mix for these recipes, you may not need to add all of it since it's a slightly larger mix.

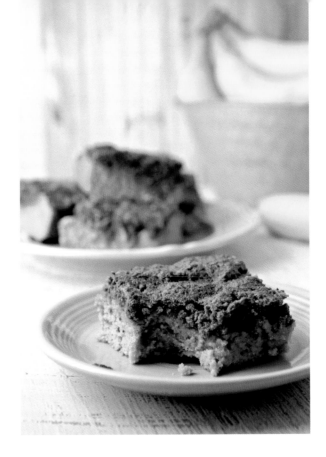

Two-Tone Banana Bars

——— WHAT YOU NEED ———

*1 recipe Sugar Cookie Mix (page
212) or Dairy-Free, Gluten-Free
Sugar Cookie Mix (page 213)*

½ cup yogurt

½ cup butter, softened

1 egg

2 bananas, mashed

¼ cup unsweetened cocoa powder

In a large bowl, combine the cookie mix, yogurt, butter, and egg. Remove 1 cup of dough and set aside. Add the mashed bananas into the large bowl and mix well. Mix the cocoa powder with the reserved dough in the small bowl. Place the banana batter into a greased 8x8-inch baking dish, drop the chocolate batter on top of the banana batter, and use a butter knife to swirl the chocolate batter into the banana batter. Bake at 350 degrees for 35 to 40 minutes or until a toothpick inserted in the center of the bars comes out clean. Cool and cut into bars.

For a dairy-free version, replace the butter with coconut butter and the yogurt with a dairy-free alternative.

Fruity Sugar Cookie Bars

——————— WHAT YOU NEED ———————

1 recipe Sugar Cookie Mix (page
212) or Dairy-Free, Gluten-Free
Sugar Cookie Mix (page 213)
½ cup butter, melted

½ cup sour cream or yogurt
1 egg
1 jar (10 to 12 ounces) fruit preserves

In a large bowl, mix together the cookie mix, butter, sour cream, and egg. Press half of the dough into a greased 8x8-inch baking dish. Spread a layer of fruit preserves over the top of the dough. Top with the remaining dough and spread into as even a layer as possible. Bake at 350 degrees for 40 minutes or until the dough is baked through. Cut into bars and serve warm or cooled.

For a dairy-free version, replace the butter with coconut butter and the sour cream with full-fat coconut milk.

Fruit "Pizza"

——————— WHAT YOU NEED ———————

1 recipe Sugar Cookie Mix (page
212) or Dairy-Free, Gluten-Free
Sugar Cookie Mix (page 213)
1 egg
½ cup sour cream or yogurt

½ cup butter, melted
12 ounces cream cheese, softened
1 tablespoon sugar
1 tablespoon vanilla extract
Diced fresh fruit

In a large bowl, combine the cookie mix, egg, sour cream, and butter. Roll out the dough onto a greased large rectangular cookie sheet or pizza pan. Bake at 350 degrees for 10 minutes or until golden brown. In another bowl, mix together the softened cream cheese, sugar, and vanilla extract until smooth and spread evenly over the cooled crust. Top the pizza with diced pieces of your favorite fruits. Strawberries and blueberries are some of our favorites!

Money-Saving Tip: Save the desserts for a few times a week and special occasions. We usually only make dessert or cookies once or twice a week to keep our sugar intake to a minimum. Desserts can often have more expensive ingredients as well, so cutting back on desserts will be healthy for your budget too!

hot chocolate mix

. . .

I'll admit, in the winter I'm a hot chocolate fanatic. Because of my allergies, I can't drink coffee, but I still want a nice warm drink now and then to warm my belly, and tea doesn't count—sometimes you just NEED chocolate! I've seen many variations of hot chocolate mix recipes but this is our favorite. It is very simple and frugal. A cup of hot chocolate using this mix costs only pennies.

Of course, around the holidays, this mix also makes a great gift. Package some in a cute little jar tied with a pretty red or green ribbon and you are good to go. This mix makes a great gift for your friends who have food allergies since it's free of most common allergens and can be made with a nondairy milk.

—————— WHAT YOU NEED ——————

1 teaspoon sea salt
1⅓ cups raw sugar (brown sugar will work)
2 cups unsweetened cocoa powder

Toss the salt and sugar together in the blender and blend until they are powdered. Mix in the cocoa powder. Store the mix in a jar or container until ready to use.

To make hot chocolate, simply mix 1 heaping tablespoon of mix into a mug of warm milk or filtered water. You can use coconut or almond milk if you are dairy-free. Stir until blended and enjoy! Top with whipped cream if desired.

If you want a gourmet hot chocolate, there are many fun things you can add to your drink. Here are some ideas to get you inspired!

- A sprinkle of Vanilla Sugar (page 220)
- A pinch of cinnamon
- A few chocolate chips
- A drizzle of maple syrup

Money-Saving Tip: Always shop with a grocery list and stick to it. Adding extras to your cart just takes away from your hard-earned grocery budget, and often impulse purchases aren't the healthiest choices. Also make sure to shop when you aren't hungry (right after breakfast is a good time because you have just eaten and because grocery stores tend to discount meats and other items in the early morning), and shop alone if at all possible.

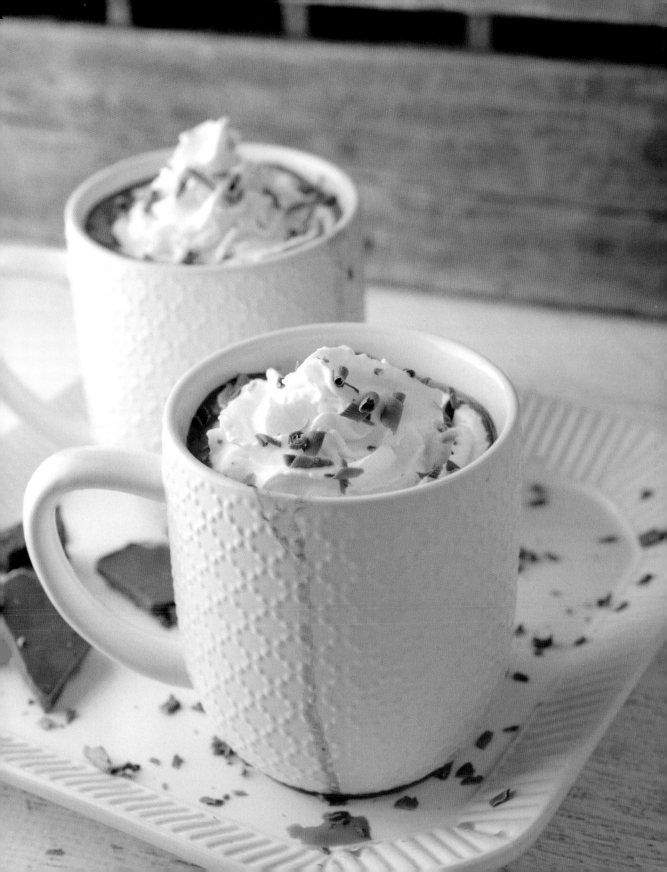

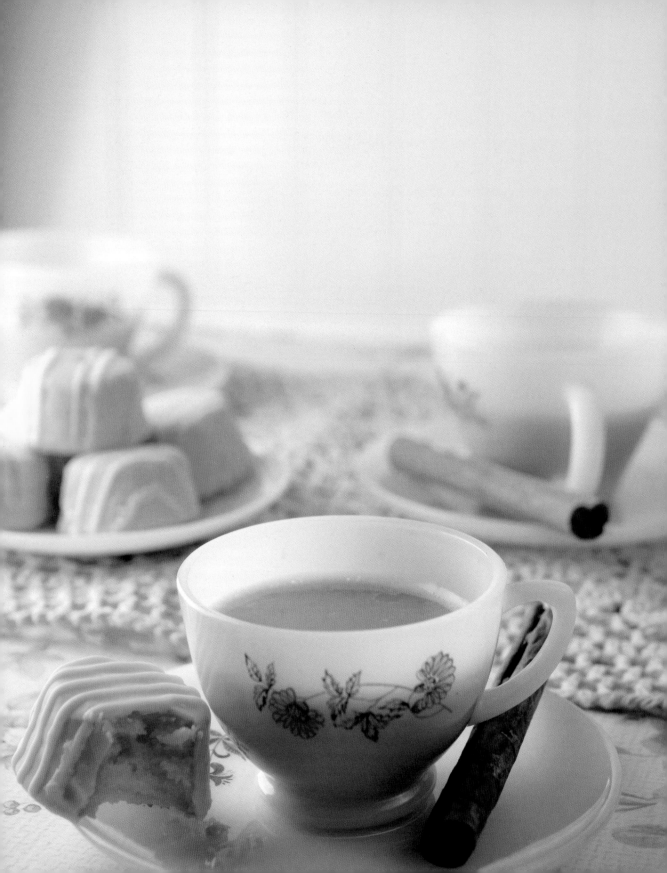

chai tea mix

. . .

I remember learning what this drink was when I was in high school. I thought it was such a fancy, special drink. Coffee shops and specialty drinks were just starting to become really popular during that time. Of course, my frugal mom had to show me that we didn't need a coffee shop to make a fancy drink; we could simply make it ourselves at home, and better yet, make a mix version so we could enjoy it whenever we wanted! So here's a chai tea mix for when you need a "fancy" drink. This mix also makes a great gift for your fancy friends!

———————— WHAT YOU NEED ————————

2½ cups sugar
2 teaspoons ground ginger
2 teaspoons cinnamon
1 teaspoon ground cloves
1 teaspoon ground cardamom

Combine all the ingredients together in a food processor or blender and process until powdery. Store the mix in a jar or container.

To make chai tea, simply brew a cup of your favorite black or green tea and add 1 to 2 teaspoons of mix to your mug, plus a bit of milk. Stir well and enjoy!

As with the Hot Chocolate Mix, you can use nondairy milk (such as coconut or almond milk) to keep it dairy-free. Nondairy milk will also add a bit of extra flavor!

Money-Saving Tip: Need to save money on your grocery bill? Try a one-week-long Eat from the Pantry Challenge. Eat only things that you already have in your pantry and freezer and do not step foot in a store all week. You might just find that you can be quite creative in the kitchen when challenged to use what you have on hand!

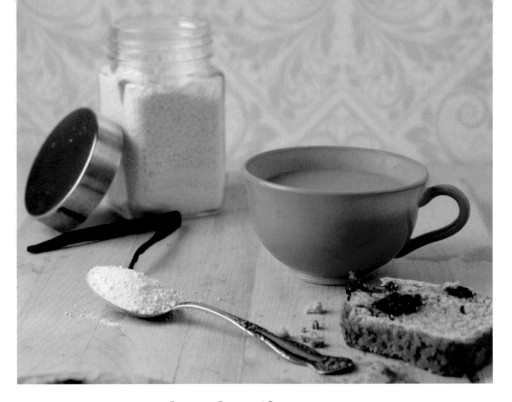

powdered coffee creamer

· · ·

You can easily skip the store-bought version of coffee creamer, which can cost several dollars a bottle and taste a little bit like plastic.

I'm not a coffee drinker, but my husband is, and a picky one at that. I once bought him some creamer that I thought looked good and was even semi "healthy." All that creamer did was sit in my fridge until it finally curdled and ended up in my pig slop pail! But even he approves of my recipe for homemade powdered coffee creamer. And I love this recipe because it's very, very easy.

For this recipe you will not want to use vanilla extract, because even though it smells amazing, it will taste bitter in your drink. Making vanilla sugar is quite easy, though you will have to do it ahead of time in order to have it ready for this recipe.

Vanilla Sugar

WHAT YOU NEED

2 cups sugar
1 whole vanilla bean

Split the vanilla bean open with a sharp knife. Scrape the contents into the sugar, then cut up the bean into a few large pieces and put it in with the sugar as well. Let the flavors develop in an airtight container for 1 to 2 weeks. After that time, remove the bean pieces and give the sugar a stir. You can then use it in coffee creamer or to flavor other drinks and treats.

Coffee Creamer

———————— WHAT YOU NEED ————————

2 cups Vanilla Sugar
8 cups powdered milk or powdered coconut milk
2 tablespoons coconut oil (optional)

Mix the vanilla sugar and powdered milk together. In a food processor or blender, process into a powder. If using coconut oil, place the mixture in a bowl and pour the coconut oil over the top and mix it in thoroughly. (If you want to make sure your coffee does not have a coconut flavor but you want the richness that the coconut oil adds, make sure to use an expeller-pressed coconut oil.)

Put the entire mixture in a large container and use as a coffee creamer as needed.

This recipe will last at least a month (longer if stored in the fridge). You can always make extra vanilla sugar at one time (since that's the longest part of the process for making this creamer) and have it ready for your next batch.

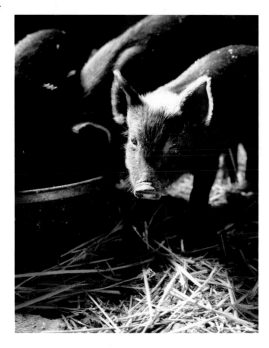

Money-Saving Tip: Watch for food waste. Make sure that all leftovers from meals get eaten, and if something is too large to get eaten up quickly, freeze it for later. In our house we have a "leftover buffet" where we get out all the leftovers from the fridge once a week and set them out buffet-style to enjoy for a meal. You get a little taste of everything, and all the leftovers get used up!

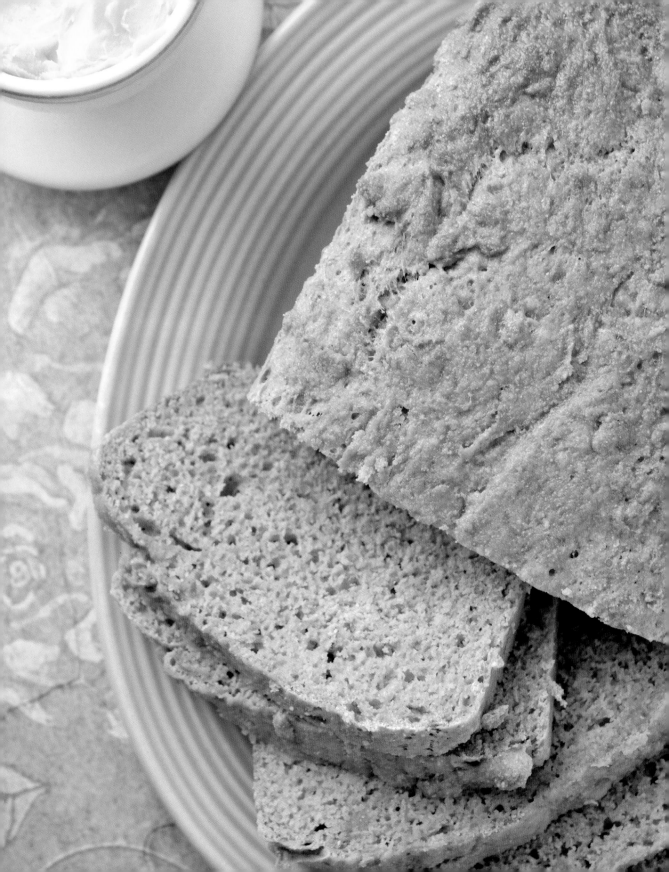

homemade basic breads

· · ·

Sometimes you need a shortcut for your shortcut! Baking bread in our bread machine is already the less time-consuming way to go, but something else that we've found saves time is simply to have the dry ingredients already mixed up and ready to go.

This recipe makes a simple bread and is the perfect size for any two-pound bread machine. If your bread machine is smaller than two pounds, just cut this recipe in half.

Bread Machine Mix

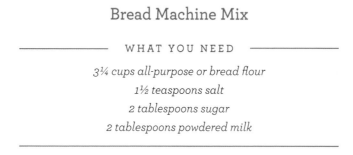

─────── WHAT YOU NEED ───────

3¼ cups all-purpose or bread flour
1½ teaspoons salt
2 tablespoons sugar
2 tablespoons powdered milk

Mix all the ingredients together until well blended. Store in a jar or storage bag until ready to use.

Bread Machine Bread

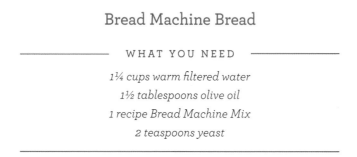

─────── WHAT YOU NEED ───────

1¼ cups warm filtered water
1½ tablespoons olive oil
1 recipe Bread Machine Mix
2 teaspoons yeast

In your bread machine, first add the water and oil. Pour the bread mix on top and make a little indentation in the mix to place the yeast in. Set your machine on the bread setting (or whatever setting will mix the dough and bake the bread) and let it do its job.

You can also substitute whole wheat flour for the white flour in this recipe or use half white and half wheat.

Handmade Bread Mix

If you are looking to make homemade bread, you can always use the same recipe as the bread machine recipe and just knead it yourself (and let it rise) and bake it in the oven for a handmade version. But I prefer to make a few loaves when I make home-made bread, since it tends to take some time. Any loaves we don't eat right away, I simply place in the freezer for a fresh-made bread that we can pull out at any time.

There really isn't much in bread, it's just the kneading and rising that take some time, and having a few ingredients already mixed up will help shave a few minutes off your day and hopefully help create less mess in the kitchen.

————— ——— WHAT YOU NEED —————

2 tablespoons sugar

1 tablespoon salt

6 cups all-purpose flour, bread flour, or whole wheat flour

½ cup powdered milk

Mix all the ingredients together well. Store in a jar or storage bag until ready to make bread.

Handmade Bread

————— WHAT YOU NEED —————

2 cups lukewarm filtered water

2 teaspoons yeast

2 tablespoons butter, melted

1 recipe Bread Mix

In a small bowl, mix together 1 cup of the lukewarm water and the yeast. Let it sit until the yeast is foamy (about 5 minutes). If for some reason your yeast doesn't foam, try it again. If you still do not have luck, you may want to pick up another package of yeast at the store because yours may be too old. In a large bowl, mix the other cup of lukewarm water and the butter. Add the yeast mixture and begin adding the bread mix. First blend half the mix into the dough. Once that is combined, add the rest.

Knead the dough by pushing it down and folding it over at least 10 times. Let it rise, covered with a clean towel in a warm area, for about 45 minutes. Punch the dough down and grease two loaf pans. Shape the dough to fit into the loaf pans, place in the pans, and let rise another 30 minutes. Bake at 350 degrees for at least 1 hour or until the bread has become a nice brown on the top and has a slightly hollow sound when tapped.

When you remove the bread from the oven, top with a bit of melted butter to keep the crust from getting hard.

If you want to freeze one of the loaves of bread for later (homemade bread will spoil within about a week if not eaten), simply place it in a freezer storage bag or wrap with plastic and freezer paper after baking. When needed, remove from the freezer and let it thaw on the counter (in the bag) during the day; it will be ready for dinnertime. Use as you would a fresh loaf of bread.

For a fun and simple variation, top the loaves with a bit of shredded cheddar cheese just before baking.

Money-Saving Tip: Bread is something so simple that can save your household so much money. A loaf of bread at the store will cost a few dollars and the homemade version is just a few pennies. Save time by baking more than one loaf at a time and freezing the unused loaves until ready to use.

corn bread mix

. . .

Corn has been an odd thing in our household. For several years it wasn't present in any form, as our older son and I had intolerances to it. However, after several years of eating a better diet, we were able to add it back into our regular diet as long as it was organic or non-GMO corn. This opened up our menu plan for great new possibilities such as corn tortillas, corn as a simple side dish, and of course, yummy corn bread!

This corn bread mix is easy and simple. We like to use it not only for corn bread to go with soups and other dishes but also as a base for a few other recipes that I list for you. Enjoy!

─────────── WHAT YOU NEED ───────────

1 cup + 2 tablespoons cornmeal
1 cup all-purpose flour
½ cup powdered milk
¾ teaspoon salt
1 tablespoon sugar
2 teaspoons baking powder
½ teaspoon baking soda

Mix all the ingredients together well and pour into a jar or storage bag.

Corn Bread

─────────── WHAT YOU NEED ───────────

1 recipe Corn Bread Mix
½ cup butter, softened
2 eggs
¼ cup milk

Mix all the ingredients thoroughly and pour into a greased 8x8-inch baking dish. Bake at 375 degrees for 35 minutes.

If you are dairy-free, you can leave out the powdered milk completely and substitute ¾ cup nondairy milk and ¼ cup coconut oil for the butter and milk in the final recipe.

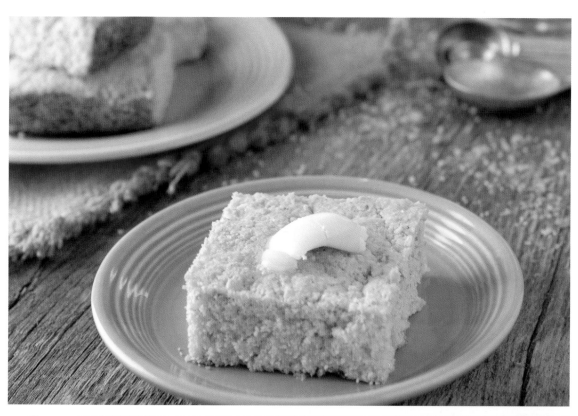
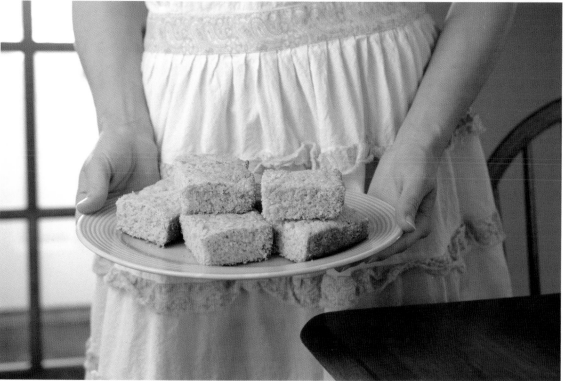

Cherry Cobbler

———————— WHAT YOU NEED ————————

1 recipe Corn Bread Mix (page 226)
4 tablespoons butter, diced into small pieces
½ cup milk
3 tablespoons sugar
4 cups frozen cherries
1 cup frozen peaches

In a bowl, mix together the corn bread mix, butter, milk, and sugar until crumbly. Thaw the cherries and peaches (you can use other fruit if those aren't available) and pour into a 9x13-inch baking dish. Sprinkle the corn bread crumble over the top. Bake at 350 degrees for 40 minutes or until the fruit layer is bubbly. Serve with ice cream.

For a dairy-free version, leave out the powdered milk in the corn bread mix, replace the milk with a nondairy milk such as almond or coconut milk, and replace the butter with coconut butter.

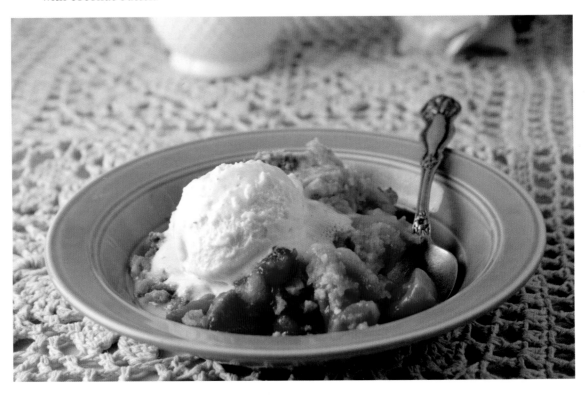

Corndog Bites

WHAT YOU NEED

1 recipe Corn Bread Mix (page 226)
½ cup butter, melted
¼ cup milk
2 eggs
8 uncured, nitrate-free hot dogs

Grease a mini muffin tin. Mix up the corn bread mix, butter, milk, and eggs and place a small amount into each muffin tin pocket. Cut the hot dogs into small pieces, about ½ to ¾ inch long, and place on top of the batter. (If you are using nitrate-free hot dogs, make sure they are cooked first!) Pour more batter over the top of the hot dogs until all of the pockets are three-quarters full. Bake at 350 degrees for about 15 minutes.

For Corndog Muffins, make these in a regular muffin pan.

For a dairy-free version, leave out the powdered milk in the corn bread mix, replace the butter with coconut oil, and replace the milk with a dairy-free alternative.

Cheesy Corn Bread Flatbread

WHAT YOU NEED

1 recipe Corn Bread Mix (page 226)
2 cups milk
1 tablespoon olive oil
2 cups shredded cheddar cheese, divided

In a large bowl, combine the corn bread mix, milk, olive oil, and 1 cup of the cheddar cheese. Pour half of the mixture into a greased 9x13-inch pan and sprinkle with half of the remaining cheese. Bake for 25 minutes at 350 degrees and cool. Remove from the pan and repeat, using the rest of the batter and cheese (you can make a single batch by using only half the mix and cutting the rest of the recipe in half). Cut into pieces when cool and use for sandwich bread or just for a side dish.

Money-Saving Tip: Found an anthill? Sprinkle some cornmeal around the hill and watch the ants go away. Ants cannot digest cornmeal, so it's an easy solution to get them to move out!

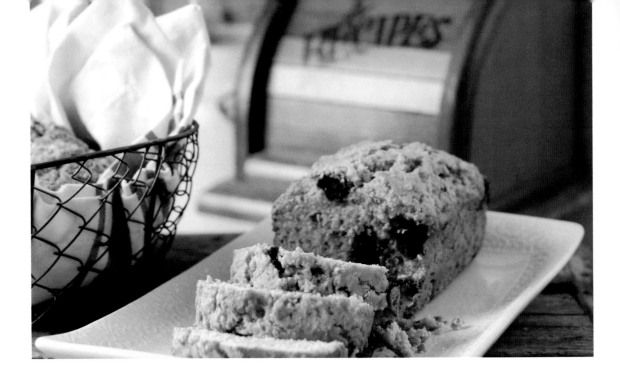

quick bread mix

· · ·

It's always great to have a mix on hand to make your favorite little loaves when you need them. Quick breads are versatile—great for breakfasts, desserts, and snacks or as a side dish to your meal.

We love this recipe because it makes a quick bread base and is adaptable to many different flavors depending on what we are feeling like at the time.

One recipe makes enough for one loaf of bread, so double or triple up if you plan to make several loaves at a time. I have a mini loaf pan that holds four loaves at one time. I like to bake several batches and give one of the little loaves to our neighbors as a special treat from our home to theirs.

———————— WHAT YOU NEED ————————

2 cups all-purpose flour or All-Purpose Gluten-Free Flour Mix (page 164)
½ cup sugar
2 teaspoons baking powder
1 teaspoon salt

Mix all the ingredients thoroughly and store in a jar or storage bag until ready to use.

Quick Bread

─────── WHAT YOU NEED ───────

1 recipe Quick Bread Mix

1 egg

1 cup milk (use 1 cup with dry add-ins or ½ cup

with wet add-ins like fruits)

2 tablespoons butter, melted

Add-ins (see below)

Mix together all the ingredients until thoroughly combined. Pour into a greased loaf pan and bake at 350 degrees for about 45 minutes or until a toothpick inserted into the center of the loaf comes out clean.

For a dairy-free quick bread, replace the milk with a nondairy milk such as almond or coconut milk and replace the butter with coconut butter.

Money-Saving Tip: Banana bread is one of our favorite quick breads, but instead of tossing the peels after adding the banana into the mix, I throw them into the garden. Banana peels make an excellent healthy compost for your soil. If you want to make a good plant booster, dry the banana peels and create a powder. Place this powder around your plants whenever they need a boost.

Quick Bread Add-in Ideas

1 mashed banana

1 large finely diced apple

1 cup shredded zucchini

2 mashed pears

½ cup dried cherries

½ cup diced dried apricots

½ cup blueberries

½ cup chocolate chips

½ cup nuts or coconut

cobbler mix

· · ·

We love making cobblers at any time of year. In the summer and fall there is always an abundance of fresh fruit just waiting to be cobblered, and in the winter we use frozen or canned fruit that we have put away. My favorite way to make cobbler is in the slow cooker. All I have to do is add a few ingredients and let them cook for a few hours, and we have a delicious dessert to go with our meal! I love this method of cooking cobbler, especially in the summer, since it doesn't heat up the kitchen the way letting the oven run does.

To make my recipe for cobbler even simpler, I like to mix up the dry ingredients ahead of time and store them in my pantry. This way, when I'm ready to make the cobbler, instead of having to pull out several ingredients and measure them all out, I can just pull a jar of Cobbler Mix off the pantry shelf and pour it in. It makes an already easy dessert even easier to make!

To make this more time-effective, you may want to make several of these at a time and fill your pantry shelf.

──────── WHAT YOU NEED ────────

1 cup all-purpose flour or
All-Purpose Gluten-Free Flour Mix (page 164)
⅓ cup brown sugar
⅓ cup uncooked old-fashioned oats

Mix all the ingredients together and pour into a ziplock bag, container, or glass jar. These amounts are enough to make one mix.

Cobbler

──────── WHAT YOU NEED ────────

4 cups fresh, canned, or frozen fruit
brown sugar (optional)
1 recipe Cobbler Mix
1 stick butter (½ cup)

Chop the fruit into pieces. We like to use apples, pears, peaches, strawberries, or a mixture such as apples and pears or strawberry and rhubarb. Unless your fruit is canned, you might want to add a little sugar into the chopped fruit so it's not too sour. I add about ¼ cup of brown sugar per every 4 cups of fruit.

Pour the fruit into a 3-quart slow cooker. If you are using a larger slow cooker, you may want to double the recipe. Pour the cobbler mix on top of the fruit and spread it so it's even. Melt the stick of butter and pour on top of the mixture. Use a fork and poke the butter into the mixture. Cook for 4 hours on the low setting, or until bubbly. Enjoy warm. For a treat, top with a scoop of ice cream.

For a dairy-free version, replace the butter with coconut butter.

Money-Saving Tip: Fruit can be so expensive out of season. Make fruit desserts and side dishes by creatively using whatever fruits happen to be in season at the time or going for frozen fruits when fresh is not available at a fair price. When you buy fruits in season, you will not only save money but also get your family to try new things and expand their horizons. Buying and trying fruit this way recently got our family to love apricots, which then led to our planting some apricot trees around the yard. We didn't even know we liked them until we bought them in season and found a great deal on them!

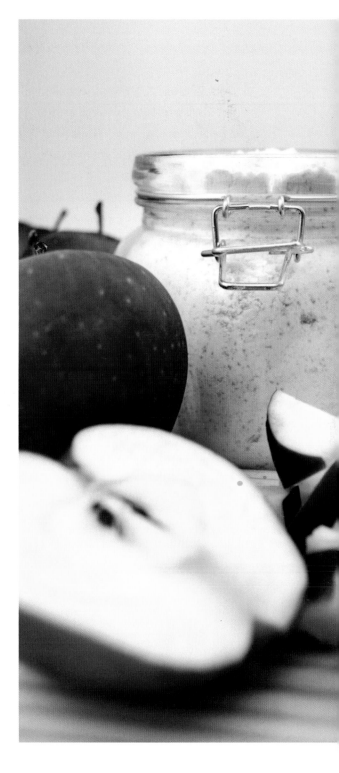

instant refried beans

. . .

Beans are one of the best inexpensive dishes you can create. Dried beans cost only a few dollars or less per bag and they make a good amount of food when cooked. Plus they are full of protein! The only bad thing about using dried beans in recipes and for meals is that they take a long time to cook. That's why you need this recipe for Instant Refried Beans and why it will become a pantry staple in your household!

First you will need to create bean powder. The best beans to use in this recipe are navy or pinto beans or a mixture of both. To do this you don't want to simply grind up beans. Beans are covered with what's called "field dust," dirt from the field, dirt from transportation, and anything else that landed on the beans in between. Give your dried beans a good rinse (you can use your homemade Produce Wash Spray, page 91) and lay them out on a clean kitchen towel to dry. Make sure they dry overnight or for a long length of time to ensure that they are very dry before grinding.

To grind beans, simply place a small amount (about 1 cup at a time) in a food processor, blender, (clean) coffee grinder, or flour mill and grind to a powder. A blender will work, but just keep in mind that it may wear your blender out more quickly, as dry goods can be hard on the motor. For the sake of convenience, I usually go with a blender, but for a large amount I prefer to use my flour mill. Grind a total of 3 cups of beans per recipe.

--- WHAT YOU NEED ---

3 cups ground dried beans

2 teaspoons salt

1 tablespoon onion powder

1 teaspoon garlic powder

2 teaspoons chili powder

Mix all the ingredients together and store in a quart jar or large ziplock bag until ready to use.

To rehydrate the beans for a quick meal or to add to ground beef to stretch it, you will need:

2½ cups filtered water

¾ cup Instant Refried Beans

1 tablespoon butter or coconut oil

(extra-virgin if possible)

Heat the water until boiling and add the refried bean powder and butter. Stir until the mixture becomes thick and is combined with the water.

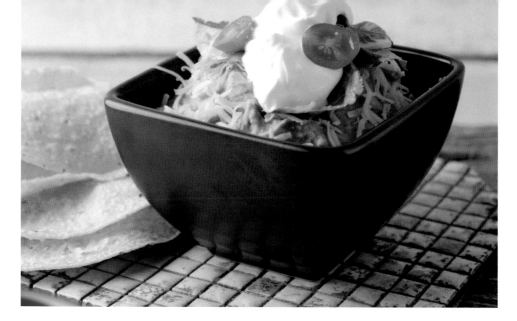

Quick Bean Bowls

For a quick lunch, we make up the Instant Refried Beans as detailed on page 234, then add shredded cheese, rice, cilantro, salsa, lettuce, diced tomatoes, and sour cream on top.

Bean Dip

──────────────── WHAT YOU NEED ────────────────

¾ cup Instant Refried Beans
(page 234)
1 tablespoon butter
2½ cups filtered water
1 jalapeño, diced

1 tablespoon vinegar
½ teaspoon sugar
¼ teaspoon paprika
¼ teaspoon cayenne powder

In a saucepan, mix together the refried bean powder, the butter, and the water. Simmer until beans are rehydrated. Add the jalapeño and simmer a bit longer. Remove from heat and add the remaining ingredients. Serve with tortilla chips.

Money-Saving Tip: Beans are a healthy, frugal staple that can easily be incorporated into your meal plans. If your family likes beans, you could replace one meat meal with beans each week; if they don't, try adding them into soups or hamburger meat by pureeing them and mixing them in. They will make the meat taste moister and your family probably won't even know they're there. This is how I got my husband to start eating beans!

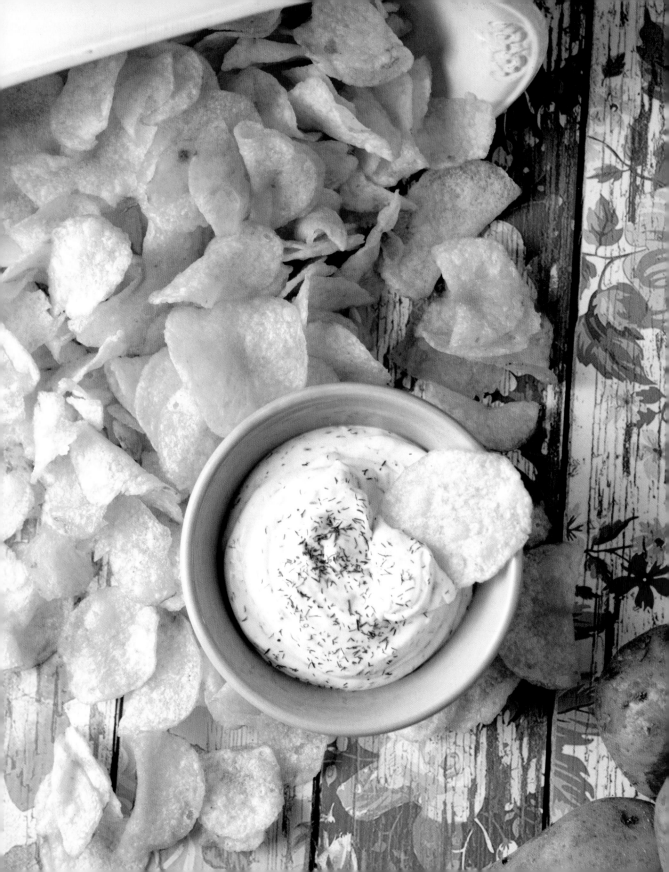

homemade dip mixes

. . .

If my little ones decide they don't want to eat their veggies, they can usually be persuaded with some dip to put them in! Here are a few dip mixes that you'll find very useful to have in your pantry.

Dill Dip and Spread Mix

————————— WHAT YOU NEED —————————

2 cups dried dill

4 tablespoons minced onion

1 tablespoon and 1 teaspoon garlic powder

1 tablespoon and 1 teaspoon dry mustard

Mix all the ingredients together until well combined and store in a jar or storage bag until ready to use.

When you are ready to create your dip or spread, combine ½ cup of the mix with 8 ounces softened cream cheese and ½ cup sour cream until thoroughly combined. For a delicious bagel spread, omit the sour cream.

Fiesta Dip Mix

————————— WHAT YOU NEED —————————

⅓ cup dried parsley

¼ cup chili powder

¼ cup minced onion

2 tablespoons salt

1 tablespoon cumin

2 tablespoons dried chives

Mix all the ingredients together until well combined and store in a jar or storage bag until ready to use.

When you are ready to create this dip, mix 3 tablespoons of the mix with 1 cup sour cream and 1 cup mayonnaise.

Herb Dip and Spread Mix

WHAT YOU NEED

1 tablespoon and 1 teaspoon dried chives

1 tablespoon and 1 teaspoon caraway seed

1 tablespoon and 1 teaspoon dried dill

1 tablespoon and 1 teaspoon dried basil

2 teaspoons garlic powder

½ teaspoon pepper

Mix all the ingredients together until well combined and store in a jar or a storage bag until ready to use.

When you are ready to create this dip, mix 3 tablespoons of the mix with 8 ounces softened cream cheese and ½ cup sour cream. For a delicious bagel spread, omit the sour cream.

Money-Saving Tip: Herbs are very easy to grow and you can grow them year-round. Plant a few seeds in a flowerpot and place near a window or natural light and watch them grow! Harvest herbs when they are mature and dry the extras for later.

homemade seasoning mixes

. . .

There are so many advantages to homemade seasonings, but the ones I appreciate the most are that they are less expensive than the store versions and, of course, that I know exactly what is in them. There are so many different seasonings that you can create depending on what you love to cook, but these are some of our favorites. We use these in many different dishes, so it's worth creating them ahead of time to have on hand for saving time later; you can always add things as you need them for a specific recipe.

Certain spices can be more expensive to buy, but the best place we've found to purchase them is in bulk from health food stores or co-ops. You can buy exactly what you need and you will end up paying less since you don't have to pay for the packaging.

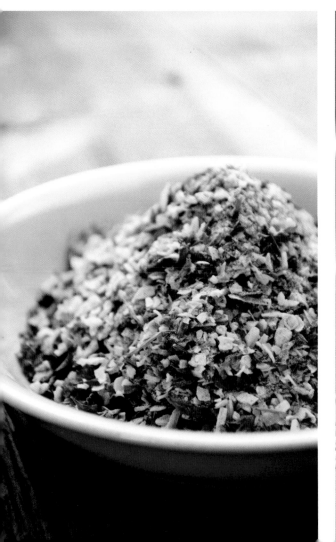
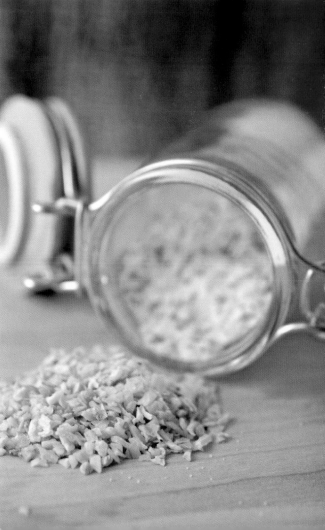

Roast Topping

I use this as a topping not only for roasts but also for steaks and other meats. It's so easy to make a meal with! Most of the time I simply place my roast or meat in the slow cooker, sprinkle with about 1 teaspoon seasoning mix per pound of meat, and cook for the rest of the day for an easy meal.

──────────── WHAT YOU NEED ────────────

1 cup minced garlic

1 cup minced onion

1 teaspoon ground black pepper

Mix all the ingredients together and store in a pint jar until needed.

Seasoning Salt

While I'm not a fan of seasoning salt, my hubby is, so this is something I like to keep on hand for him. It's very similar to the store version and can be used to season a variety of foods.

──────────── WHAT YOU NEED ────────────

1 teaspoon dried parsley

1 tablespoon celery seed

1 cup sea salt

1 tablespoon onion powder

1 teaspoon paprika

1 teaspoon chili powder

1 teaspoon garlic powder

Place the parsley and celery seed in a small blender or food processor and pulse until powdered. In a bowl, combine with the remaining ingredients until blended. Store in a pint jar.

Taco Seasoning

Taco seasoning is a basic staple in most households. We use it for everything from seasoning taco meat to making a taco dip with sour cream and cream cheese.

──────────── WHAT YOU NEED ────────────

½ cup minced onion

⅓ cup garlic salt

¼ cup chili powder

2 tablespoons cumin

3 tablespoons oregano

¼ cup cornstarch

2 teaspoons red pepper

flakes (optional)

Mix all the ingredients together and store in a pint jar. Leave the red pepper flakes out of the mixture if you prefer less heat. Use 2 tablespoons of seasoning per pound of beef.

Fajita Seasoning

Fajita seasoning is a little sweeter and has a little more heat than taco seasoning. It's perfect for seasoning meat and veggies for fajitas! We usually mix this up in a smaller amount at a time than the taco seasoning, simply because it's used less. Double the recipe if you make a lot of fajitas.

—————— WHAT YOU NEED ——————

3 tablespoons cornstarch

2 tablespoons chili powder

1 tablespoon salt

1 tablespoon sugar

2½ teaspoons Faux Bouillon

(page 177)

1½ teaspoons onion powder

½ teaspoon garlic powder

½ teaspoon cayenne pepper

¼ teaspoon red pepper flakes

½ teaspoon cumin

Mix all the ingredients together and store in a small jar. The amount you use will be based on your tastes, but estimate roughly 2 tablespoons of seasoning per pound of meat/veggies.

Herb Seasoning

This is a great all-purpose seasoning for vegetables. One favorite use for it in our house is to coat summer veggies before we toss them on the grill.

—————— WHAT YOU NEED ——————

2 teaspoons sea salt

½ teaspoon thyme

1 teaspoon basil

½ teaspoon celery seed

1 teaspoon garlic powder

1 teaspoon sage

1 teaspoon oregano

1 teaspoon onion powder

Mix all the ingredients together and store in a small jar.

Ranch Dressing Mix

This seasoning mix is a fun one to make, and it has so many different uses!

WHAT YOU NEED

5 tablespoons minced onion

1 tablespoon salt

1 teaspoon garlic powder

2 teaspoons black pepper

2½ tablespoons dried parsley

2 teaspoons paprika

1 teaspoon celery salt

In a medium bowl, mix together all the ingredients until blended. Store in a sealed container in a cool, dark place (like a pantry) until ready to use. 1 tablespoon of the mix equals 1 tablespoon of ranch dressing mix from the store.

Here are some great ways you can use this mix in your daily cooking:

Ranch Dressing

Mix 2 tablespoons of the Ranch Dressing Mix with 1 cup sour cream, 1 cup mayonnaise, and ½ cup milk. Stir together until well blended. The longer you let this sit in the fridge, the better it will taste. Pour this over salad, potatoes, chicken, pizza, wraps, sandwiches, vegetables, and more!

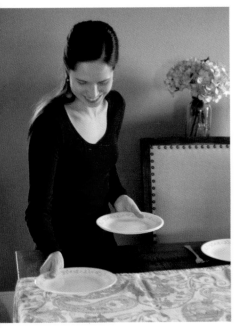

Ranch Dip

Mix 1 tablespoon of the Ranch Dressing Mix with 1 cup sour cream. Stir until well blended. Make it a few hours before you plan on serving, so the sour cream has time to soak up the flavor of the mix. Dip with your favorite chips or tortillas.

Ranch Veggies

Peel and dice 3 pounds of potatoes. Place in a large bowl with 1 teaspoon of the Ranch Dressing Mix and one tablespoon of vegetable oil and toss until well coated. Bake in an oven at 400 degrees for 30 minutes or until the potatoes are cooked through. You can also add other veggies (carrots, onions, peppers) to this dish.

Italian Seasoning

Yet another staple seasoning to keep in your pantry. This one is so easy to make!

─────────── WHAT YOU NEED ───────────

2 tablespoons dried basil

2 tablespoons dried marjoram

2 tablespoons dried oregano

1 tablespoon dried sage

2 tablespoons dried thyme

2 tablespoons dried rosemary

Mix all the ingredients together until well blended and store in a small jar.

Italian Dressing Mix

This recipe uses some of the Italian Seasoning mix to make a delicious dressing.

─────────── WHAT YOU NEED ───────────

4 tablespoons garlic powder

4 tablespoons onion powder

4 tablespoons paprika

2 tablespoons + 2 teaspoons
Italian Seasoning

2 teaspoons oregano

2 teaspoons dried basil

1 tablespoon + 1 teaspoon salt

½ teaspoon pepper

Mix all the ingredients until thoroughly combined and store in a small jar.

Italian Dressing

Combine 4 tablespoons of Italian Dressing Mix with 1 cup olive oil and ⅓ cup grated Parmesan cheese. Mix thoroughly and use as a dressing for salads.

Italian Pasta Salad

Make the Italian Dressing and pour over a mixture of cooked cold pasta, cooked cubed meats, and diced veggies (peppers, cherry tomatoes, corn, peas, etc.).

Money-Saving Tip: Make sure you buy spices in bulk from your local health food store, co-op, or warehouse store. They are much cheaper by the pound and you can buy the amounts that you need so they won't go to waste.

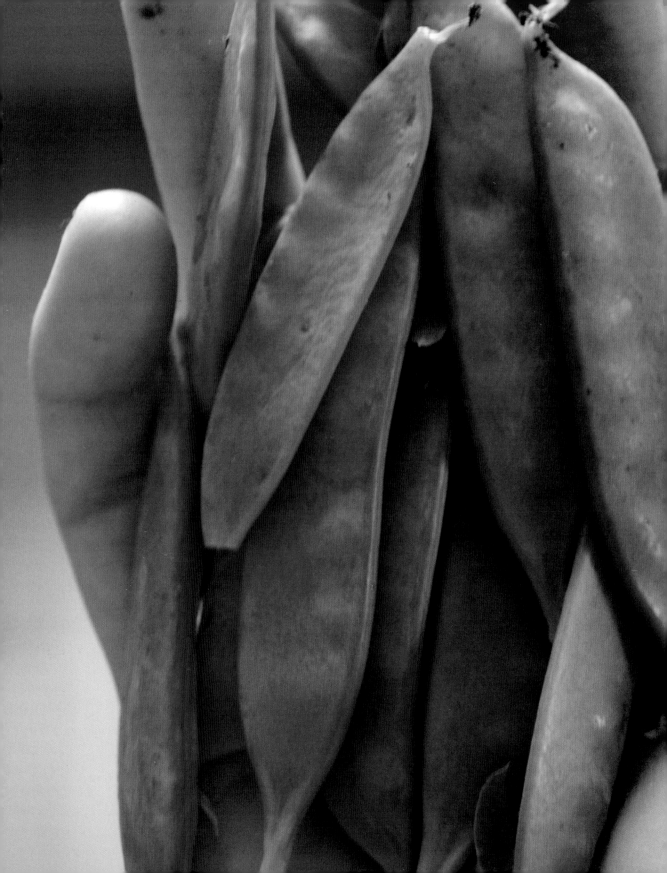

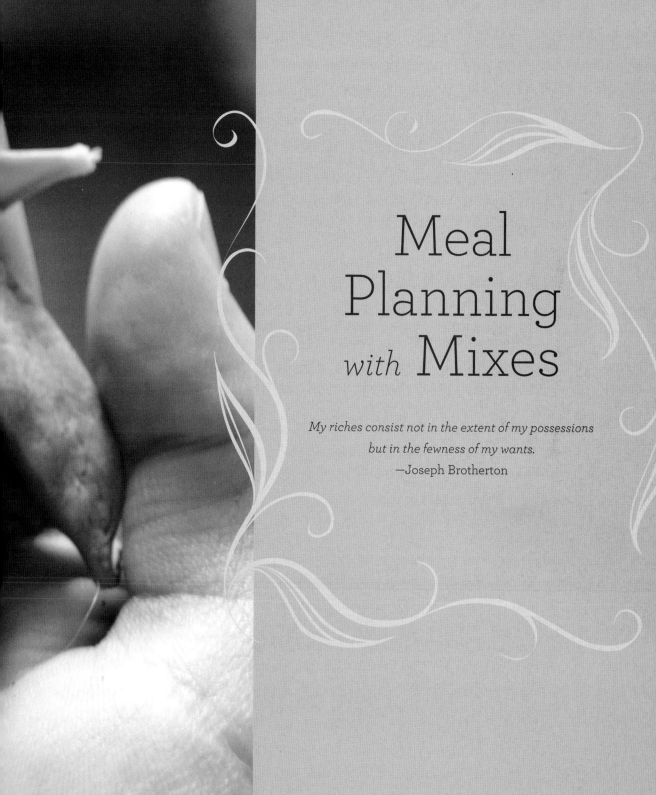

Meal
Planning
with Mixes

*My riches consist not in the extent of my possessions
but in the fewness of my wants.*
—Joseph Brotherton

Now that you have all those beautiful mixes lining your pantry, how exactly do you make meals with them? Well, unless you plan on making up a batch of brownie mix every night, there will have to be a bit of meal planning involved!

Meal planning has saved us a great deal of time and money over the last several years. It started out as a way for me to be able to tell my husband what was for dinner that night, but then I realized that it was a great help for me when I was planning my grocery shopping list, and it took a large amount of time and stress off my plate each week, since I knew exactly what I needed to do to prepare for each night's supper and I already had in my fridge and pantry what I needed to make it.

I've tried several different meal planning methods and ideas, but the one that has worked for us best is the binder method, and it's quite simple. I keep a large binder in my kitchen with all the recipes for our very favorite meals. Each week I go through the binder and pull out the recipes that I want to make that week and I move them to the front of the book and also write the list on a whiteboard that I keep on our fridge. Once I have my list of recipes I can then go through the ingredients and instructions and make a shopping list for the week.

Creating each week's meals is quite simple as well. In the morning, all I need to do is take a look at what we are having for supper that night and see if any prep work needs to be done (putting the meal in the slow cooker, getting out meat to thaw, etc.). The recipes are right there in my kitchen so I don't have to dig for them and I've already made a grocery list and shopped, so I know we have all the ingredients.

I also like to get the family involved in meal planning. Although I love to do the cooking for my family, my husband has one night a week that he plans and makes the meals. I also get the kids involved; they get to pick the veggie to go with each meal.

We created flashcards with different vegetables on them. When I write the meals on the calendar on the front of our fridge each week, I sit down with my little ones and show them the cards for the veggies that can be used as a side dish. They pick the vegetables they want and we pair them up with a meal during the week. Not only is it a great way to get them involved in something that is important in our family, it's a great way to get them excited about eating vegetables!

Once you get into the swing of it, meal planning can save so much money. You know exactly what you need to buy at the grocery store, and if you have a list it's easier to stick to it and not add extras. Plus, you know what you are going to do with what you buy, so there isn't any waste. And it can save a headache, because instead of being stuck in a rut when five o'clock rolls around, you've already got supper planned and are just working on getting it on the table.

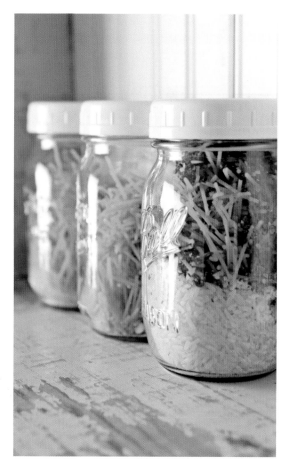

Creating homemade mixes makes meal planning and meal prepping even easier. By putting together a large part of the meals ahead, you can save some valuable time in the kitchen and still put together a full and delicious meal.

I've created a sample weekly meal plan for you using some of the mixes that you can find in this book. I hope it will spark your imagination and show you how you can add all those delicious mixes into your everyday meals!

Note: These meals are based on serving a family of four. Simply double or triple for a larger family, if your family eats a lot, or if you want to create leftovers for lunches.

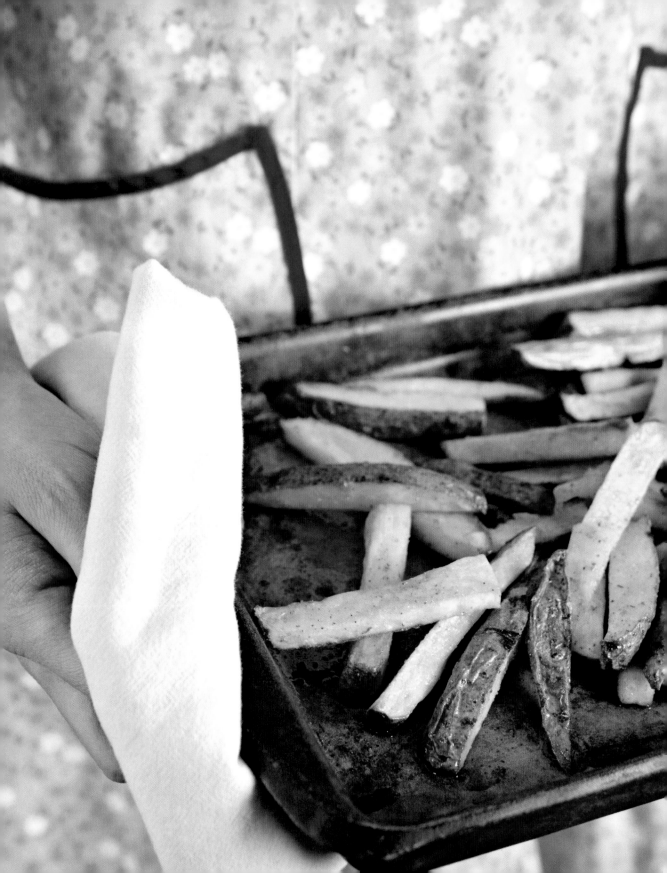

sunday

· · ·

MAIN DISH: Roast with Roast Topping

SIDE DISH: New or Fingerling Potatoes

DESSERT: Carrot Muffins

———————— WHAT YOU NEED ————————

One 3- to 4-pound roast
Roast Topping (page 240)
3 to 5 pounds new potatoes or fingerling potatoes
2¼ cups Muffin Mix (page 199)
2 eggs
1 cup milk
¼ cup butter, softened
½ cup shredded carrots
½ teaspoon cinnamon
¼ teaspoon nutmeg

What to Do

In the morning, place your roast in your slow cooker (it can be thawed or fully frozen). Add a few cups of water so the roast has something to cook in. Wash your potatoes and place them around the roast. Sprinkle the Roast Topping over the roast and potatoes and place the lid on the slow cooker. Cook on high for 6 hours and then turn to low for another 2 to 4 hours (6 to 8 hours for frozen roast). Times may depend on your slow cooker.

Make the Carrot Muffins following the instructions (page 199) about an hour before serving dinner.

monday

· · ·

MAIN DISH: Chicken with Chicken Help Mix

SIDE DISH: Green Beans

DESSERT: Peach Cobbler

——————— WHAT YOU NEED ———————

4 cups diced peaches (frozen, canned, or fresh)
Brown sugar (optional)
1 recipe Cobbler Mix (page 232)
1 stick butter (½ cup)
1 cup cooked, shredded chicken
1 recipe Chicken Help Mix (page 169)
1 cup milk
1 cup chicken broth or stock
2 cups (16 ounces) diced tomatoes
Parmesan cheese
Roughly 2 cups fresh or frozen green beans
Butter

What to Do

Around lunchtime, create a peach cobbler following the recipe instructions for the Cobbler Mix (page 232).

When you are ready to make supper, follow the instructions for Chicken Help (page 169) to create the chicken dish. When the chicken is almost ready, place the green beans in a saucepan on medium-high heat with a bit of butter. Cook them until you have them the desired consistency (some like them cooked soft and some like them crispy).

Merissa A. Alink

tuesday

. . .

MAIN DISH: Tacos with Taco Seasoning Mix

SIDE DISH: Guacamole

——————— WHAT YOU NEED ———————

1 pound ground beef

2 tablespoons Taco Seasoning (page 240)

4 to 5 avocados

½ cup salsa

Taco shells

Taco toppings (shredded cheese, sour cream,

taco sauce, salsa, etc.)

Tortilla chips

What to Do

Brown the ground beef with the Taco Seasoning. For the guacamole, simply mash the avocados and mix with the salsa. Add a bit of salt if desired. Serve with chips or add right to the tacos as an additional topping.

wednesday: breakfast for supper!

. . .

MAIN DISH: Blueberry Pancakes with Pancake Mix

SIDE DISHES: Sausage, Scrambled Eggs with Veggies

─────────── WHAT YOU NEED ───────────

1½ cups Pancake Mix (page 195)
9 eggs, divided
3 tablespoons butter
½ cup milk
½ cup fresh or frozen blueberries
Diced veggies (bell peppers, onions, tomatoes, etc.)
1 pound or package of your favorite sausage

What to Do

Mix up the pancake batter and add the blueberries, following instructions for Basic Pancakes (page 196). Scramble the remaining 8 eggs and add diced vegetables as desired. Cook the sausage until completely cooked through. (You can also cook your sausage first and then scramble the eggs in the same pan for some extra flavor!) Serve as breakfast for supper.

thursday

· · ·

MAIN DISH: Chicken Pot Pie with Baking Mix

SIDE DISH: Fruit Salad

DESSERT: Chocolate Chip Cookies with Mix

———————— WHAT YOU NEED ————————

1 cup All-Purpose Baking Mix (page 171)

1 egg

1½ cups milk or cream

2 cups diced, cooked veggies

(such as carrots, green beans, broccoli, peas, corn, etc.)

1 cup cooked, shredded chicken

¾ cup chicken stock or broth

1 teaspoon salt

1 recipe Chocolate Chip Cookie Mix (page 210)

2 eggs

1 cup butter, softened

1½ teaspoons vanilla extract

3 cups of your favorite fruits

(bananas, peaches, blueberries, strawberries, etc.)

Honey

What to Do

Mix up the Chicken Pot Pie following the recipe instructions (page 172). Mix up the cookies following the instructions for Chocolate Chip Cookies (page 210).

For the fruit salad, dice any fruit to be used (leave smaller fruits and berries like blueberries whole), drizzle with a bit of honey, and serve as a side dish.

friday

· · ·

MAIN DISH: Beef Stroganoff

SIDE DISH: Salad

———————— W H A T   Y O U   N E E D ————————

1 pound ground beef

1 cup chopped fresh mushrooms

1 recipe Beef Stroganoff Mix (page 168)

2 cups milk or beef broth or stock

½ cup sour cream

Lettuce

Salad toppings and dressing (cheese, diced fruits, nuts, etc.)

What to Do

Brown the ground beef and make the Beef Stroganoff following the recipe on page 168. Place lettuce and salad toppings on the table for a salad bar. You could also make your own Ranch Dressing (page 242) or Italian Dressing (page 243).

saturday

. . .

MAIN DISH: Chicken Breast

SIDE DISHES: Spanish Rice, Brown Sugar Baked Pears

DESSERT: Fudge Cookies

———————— WHAT YOU NEED ————————

1 pound uncooked chicken breast
1 recipe Spanish Rice Side Dish Mix (page 176)
3 cups chicken broth
4 pears
Brown sugar and butter
8 ounces cream cheese
½ cup butter, softened or melted
½ recipe Brownie Mix (page 182)

What to Do

In the morning, place the chicken breasts in the slow cooker. Add the Spanish Rice Side Dish Mix and the chicken broth. Cover and cook on high for 6 to 8 hours or until the chicken is cooked to 165 degrees on the inside when tested with a meat thermometer.

For the Brown Sugar Baked Pears, wash the pears and slice in half. Scoop out the stems and the centers and place in a greased baking dish, cut side up. Place a bit of butter inside each pear half and sprinkle with brown sugar. Bake at 350 degrees for about 15 minutes.

Mix up the cookies using the cream cheese, butter, and Brownie Mix and following the recipe on page 184.

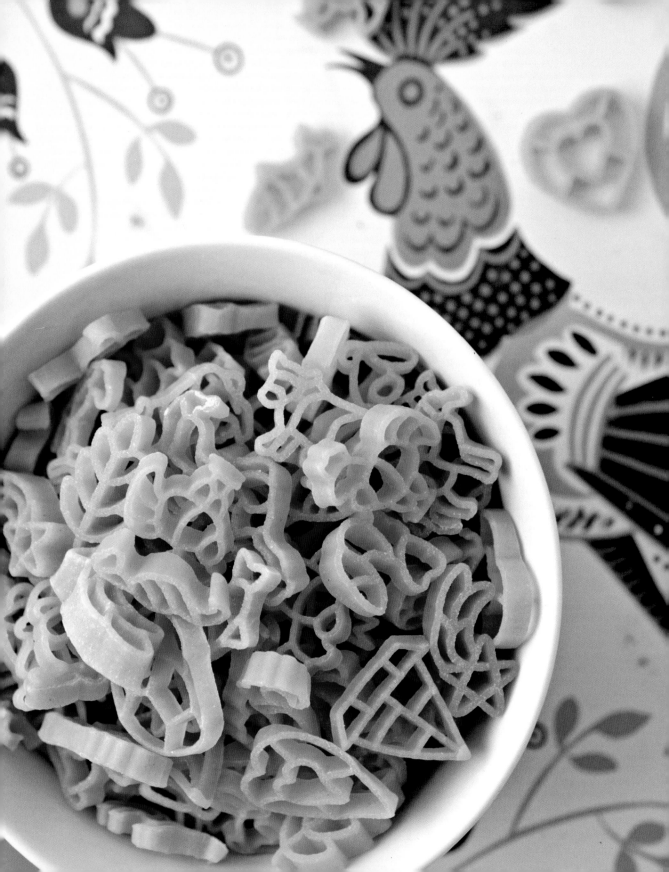

Afterword

Through our journey I've learned that happiness isn't something that just happens to us; it's something that we choose to have. There are many things we can't control in this life, but we can choose to have happiness or choose to be bitter because of our situation. Coming from the brink of losing everything, not having a dollar to our name, our many losses with food and lifestyle, and after all the hardship we've dealt with so far as a family, I have plenty of reasons to be bitter about life. But what good is that going to do me? Do my children need an unhappy mother? Does my husband need a wife who grumbles and complains all the time? Do my family and friends need someone in their lives who is always looking at the worst in every situation? Do I want to live my life as a miserable person who continually thinks, "Life isn't fair!"?

Of course not! We know that there is no way we can be happy 100 percent of the time, but looking for the light and finding the joy in every situation make us the people we know we want to be. Grateful, thoughtful living makes us an encouragement to those around us and a spark of fire in a sometimes dark world.

In the beginning I didn't understand this. It was a constant battle of "why me??" and I just couldn't figure out why I couldn't have the life we so desperately wanted—the simple life, the back-to-the-basics life. But we could have always had that life, no matter where we lived, or what our income was, and no matter what happened to be going on in our lives at that time; we just had to *choose* to have it.

Each morning when I wake up I'm thankful that I'm here. I'm thankful that I've been given my children and my husband to care for. I'm thankful that even though we might not have as nice or as many things as the Joneses, we still have each other and we have happiness and we have joy. Aren't those the things we really want in this life anyway?

If finding that kind of satisfaction is something you struggle with, I hope this book

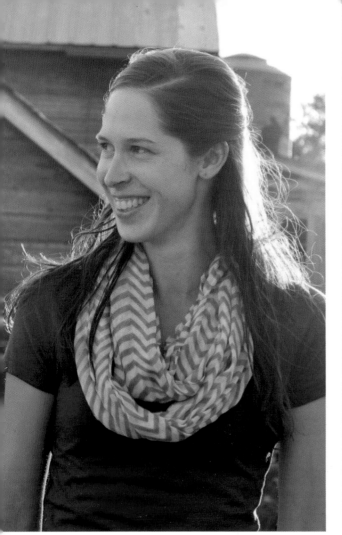
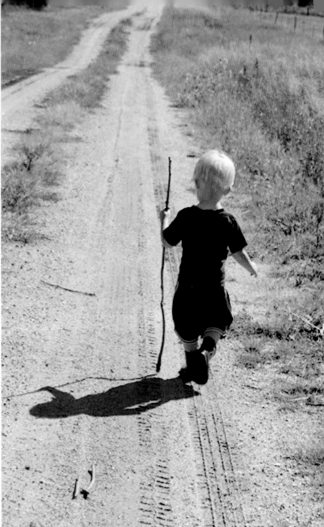

has been an encouragement to you. I hope that creating your own household and beauty products will relieve some pressure from your budget and some stress from your life. I hope that creating your own homemade mixes gives you more time to spend with your family. I hope that through some of the stories shared here, you can see that you are not alone.

Choose happiness. Choose to be the light in the darkness. Choose to make time with your family. Choose to sell some of the things in your house that are causing you clutter-stress. Choose to make a sacrifice here and there for the sake of your ultimate goals. And choose to live the best life you possibly can, no matter what your situation. Keep on keeping on and always make the most with what you have.

Appendices

Simple Substitutions

As you are creating some of the recipes in this book, you may come to realize that you don't have all the ingredients needed for the recipe. Never fear! This chapter is filled with simple substitutions for all kinds of ingredients so that you won't have to make another trip to the store.

And of course, not only does this save you a trip to the store (not to mention the time and gas spent), but you will also learn to be better prepared for any situation with the items you have on hand and become more creative in your substitutions to fit your family's dietary and allergy restrictions and needs. Something that continually frustrated me in the "allergy" recipes and cookbooks that I would read and follow was that the writer focused on only a handful of ingredients, and if you weren't able to find those, you were out of luck for the recipe. After experimenting in my own kitchen, we discovered many easy substitutions for recipes that fit not only our allergy needs but a wide variety of needs (and preferences) as well. I've included not only some substitutions that will work for the recipes in this book but a wide variety of substitutions that will work in many different recipes that you may be trying to adapt to better fit your needs and what you happen to have in the pantry at the time.

Of course, keep in mind that not every single substitution will work in every recipe that you try it in and not all substitutions have been tested in every single recipe. It will be up to you to experiment with the recipes with the ingredients that will work for you and your family. Occasionally, if you don't have the ingredients you need OR these substitutions on hand, you may actually need to make a trip to the store. I wouldn't want you attempting to try something like making sweetened condensed milk with only water and sugar, because I can assure you, that doesn't work. (Learn from my soupy, drippy, "sweetened condensed water" disaster!)

For Baking

ALLSPICE—½ teaspoon cinnamon + ½ teaspoon cloves = 1 teaspoon allspice

APPLE PIE SPICE—½ teaspoon cinnamon + ¼ teaspoon ginger + ⅛ teaspoon allspice + ⅛ teaspoon nutmeg = 1 teaspoon apple pie spice

ARROWROOT POWDER—1 tablespoon cornstarch OR 2 tablespoons flour = 1 tablespoon arrowroot

BAKING POWDER—¼ teaspoon cream of tartar + ¼ teaspoon baking soda = 1 teaspoon baking powder

BROWN SUGAR—1 cup raw sugar or Sucanat or 1 cup white sugar + 2 tablespoons molasses = 1 cup brown sugar

BUTTER—oil OR almond butter OR coconut butter

BUTTERMILK—1 cup yogurt + 1 tablespoon lemon juice or vinegar = 1 cup buttermilk

CAKE FLOUR—1 cup minus 2 tablespoons all-purpose flour (sifted) = 1 cup cake flour

CELERY SALT—¾ teaspoon salt + ¼ teaspoon celery seed = 1 teaspoon celery salt

CONFECTIONERS' SUGAR—½ cup raw sugar or Sucanat or white sugar processed in a blender with 1 tablespoon cornstarch = 1 cup confectioners' sugar

CORNSTARCH—arrowroot powder, tapioca starch, potato starch, flour

CORN SYRUP—1 cup sugar + ¼ cup of a liquid already in the recipe OR 1 cup honey = 1 cup corn syrup

CREAM—1 cup whole milk + 3 tablespoons butter = 1 cup cream or half-and-half (not for whipping)

CREAM CHEESE—cottage cheese (blended)

EGGS—1 tablespoon ground flaxseed + 1 teaspoon filtered water OR ¼ cup applesauce OR 1 mashed banana = 1 egg

EVAPORATED MILK—1 cup dry milk + 1¾ cups warm filtered water = 1 can evaporated milk

GARLIC—¼ teaspoon garlic powder = 1 clove fresh garlic

HERBS—½ teaspoon dried herbs = 1 teaspoon fresh herbs

HONEY—1¼ cups sugar + ¼ cup liquid from the recipe = 1 cup honey

LEMON JUICE—1½ teaspoons vinegar = 1 tablespoon lemon juice

MILK—⅓ cup powdered milk + 1 cup filtered water = 1 cup milk OR almond milk, coconut milk, rice milk, soy milk, hemp milk, etc.

MOLASSES—honey

ONION—1 tablespoon dried minced onion = 1 medium chopped fresh onion

POWDERED MILK—powdered goat's milk OR powdered coconut milk

POWDERED SUGAR—(*see* Confectioners' Sugar)

PUMPKIN PIE SPICE—½ teaspoon cinnamon + ¼ teaspoon ginger + ⅛ teaspoon allspice + ⅛ teaspoon nutmeg = 1 teaspoon pumpkin pie spice

RICOTTA CHEESE—cottage cheese

SHORTENING—butter

SOUR CREAM—yogurt

SWEETENED CONDENSED MILK—1 cup dry milk + ½ cup boiling filtered water + ⅔ cup sugar + 3 tablespoons melted butter, blended until smooth = 1 cup sweetened condensed milk

TAPIOCA—1½ tablespoons all-purpose flour = 1 tablespoon tapioca

VINEGAR—lemon juice

YEAST—1 package yeast OR 2 teaspoons dry active yeast = 1 yeast cake

YOGURT—sour cream OR buttermilk (*also see* Buttermilk)

For Body Products

ARROWROOT POWDER—cornstarch

AVOCADO OIL—grapeseed oil, sweet almond oil, apricot kernel oil, jojoba oil

BEESWAX—carnauba wax

BENTONITE CLAY POWDER—French green clay, fuller's earth clay

COCOA BUTTER—shea butter, kokum butter, mango butter

COCONUT OIL—olive oil, avocado oil, jojoba oil, sweet almond oil, grapeseed oil

EPSOM SALTS—coarse sea salt

VITAMIN E OIL—rosemary antioxidant extract

WITCH HAZEL—rubbing alcohol

10 Uses for Mason Jars

Mason jars come in so many sizes, you can always find the perfect size for what you need. Their main use in our house (besides canning and preserving) is for storing many of our homemade and pantry goodies. The various sizes are great for different amounts of products and they also make some very cute gift holders. Here are some other great ways that you can make use of your mason jars.

CANDLE HOLDERS. I love to pour my homemade beeswax and soy candles (pages 123–124) in mason jars because they are perfect for hot items, but they also make pretty candle holders for tea lights and votive candles. For a simple decoration, simply place the candle in the jar, set on a flat surface, and light your candle. For something fun and different you can use pretty tissue paper or even fall leaves and paint a clear coat of glue sealant under and over the top of the paper or leaves. Let it dry before using.

SOAP DISPENSERS. I only have two sinks in my house, but each of them has a cute little mason jar soap dispenser by it. You can purchase a pump kit from several online retailers, and I've seen them in a few small specialty shops. I love them as soap dispensers because they are easy to clean off when they get dirty or full of soap, and as long as you keep the pumps clean they will last a very long time.

HERB KEEPER. Place a paper towel and a small amount of water in the bottom of the jar and place your fresh herbs so the cut section of the plants sits in the water at the bottom of the jar. Place a plastic lid on the jar and store the herbs in the fridge.

TABLETOP VASE. This is another way we use them in our house every day! I have several half-gallon mason jars in various places in my dining room as vases. They are pretty and let me change up the décor as needed. They never go out of style!

MAKE AN "I LOVE YOU" JAR. One year for a gift for my husband, I took little pieces of paper each day for a year and wrote on them things that I loved about him. I placed them all in the jar and gave them to him on his birthday. You could use this same concept for many types of gifts. We also have done a Thankfulness Jar for Thanksgiving: we write down little things that each family member does that we are thankful for, and then we read them to each other at the dinner table.

SPARE CHANGE JAR. Pennies saved do add up. Use a mason jar as a piggy bank to collect any spare change from your pockets (or from your laundry). We use our spare change jars to save up for vacation.

LEFTOVER PAINT STORAGE. Have extra paint from a project or painting a room? Just pour it in a mason jar with an airtight lid. On the lid of the jar make sure to write the name and brand of the color. No more storing huge paint cans, and you can see the color through the glass.

SNACK CONTAINER. The jelly-size mason jars are the perfect size for a little snack! Just toss in your favorite snack, close the jar with a plastic screw-on lid (that you can purchase separately from the jars—great for storage!), and toss in your car or in your bag for a quick snack to grab when you are out and about.

PLANT HOLDER. I love to have green veggies growing year-round, even through the winter. To accomplish this, I keep a "winter garden" in the house. I plant various types of plants (peppers, tomatoes, etc.) in some dirt inside a jar or a container and let them grow to make some yummy fresh food for us throughout even the coldest seasons of the year. This is a great way to grow fresh herbs right on your kitchen counter as well!

SINGLE-SERVE SMOOTHIE CONTAINER. Most quart-size mason jars will fit on the base of your blender, so you can use them for single-serving size smoothies! Place your smoothie ingredients right in the jar, unscrew the blender base from the pitcher, place the blender blade onto the mouth of the mason jar, screw the base on tightly as a lid, securely attach it to the blender, and blend until smooth.

13 Uses for Baking Soda

I love keeping a huge container of baking soda on hand in my pantry at all times just because it's so incredibly useful! Baking soda costs just around $0.50 per pound or less and one pound can go a long way. Besides using it in many of the recipes in this book, here are an additional thirteen uses for that box of baking soda in your pantry.

CREATE YOUR OWN TOOTHPASTE. Mix ½ cup baking soda with ½ cup coconut oil. Use as you would a regular toothpaste.

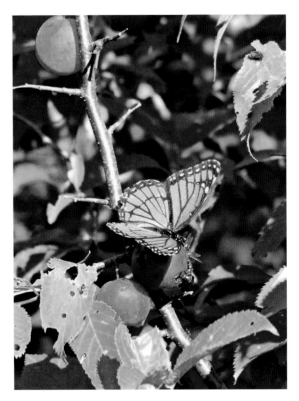

USE AS A DEODORANT IN A PINCH. Use some kind of powder puff to apply baking soda directly as a deodorant.

RELIEVE BEE STINGS BY MIXING A BIT OF BAKING SODA WITH WATER TO CREATE A PASTE. Place over the sting location to take the bite out of the sting.

ABSORB TRASH CAN ODORS. In a small bowl, mix a bit of baking soda with a few drops of your favorite essential oil. Sprinkle in the bottom of your trash can the next time you take out the trash and it will help absorb any odors.

KEEP YOUR FLOWERS FRESH. Add a bit of baking soda to the water in a vase to help keep your flowers fresher longer.

KEEP THE BUNNIES AWAY. Sprinkle a bit of baking soda around the edges of your gardens and flower beds to help repel rabbits.

SHINE YOUR STAINLESS STEEL COOKWARE. This is one of my favorite uses! Make a paste with baking soda and water and spread it over the dirty, crusted-on foods in your stainless steel cookware. Let this paste sit for up to an hour and then scrub off.

MAKE YOUR BEANS MORE DIGESTIBLE. Add just a bit of baking soda in with your water when you are soaking dried beans to help make them easier on your stomach. Make sure to rinse off all the water that the beans were soaked in before cooking.

MAKE FLUFFY EGGS. The secret to frying fluffy scrambled eggs is to add a bit of baking soda! Stir ½ teaspoon baking soda into 3 eggs that you are scrambling.

CLEAN THE FRIDGE. The next time you clean the shelves and drawers in your fridge, add a bit of baking soda to warm water and wash down the shelves and drawers to keep them clean and odor-free.

CLEAR A CLOGGED DRAIN. We've used this method many times! Sprinkle some baking soda down into a clogged drain, follow the baking soda with some vinegar, and let it bubble up in the chemical reaction. Pour very hot water down into the drain after this cleaning to make sure it's fully declogged. Repeat as needed.

GET THE BUGS OFF YOUR CAR WINDSHIELD. When regular windshield wash won't cut it, make a paste with baking soda and water and scrub onto your windshield. Let the paste sit for several minutes and lightly scrub off with more water until the bugs are removed.

CLEAN YOUR FINGERNAILS. Create a scrubbing liquid by adding a bit of hydrogen peroxide to baking soda. Use a damp cloth or a small sponge to scrub the mixture onto your fingernails to revive a healthy glow. Rinse off with water.

9 Uses for Honey

Honey is a sweet little powerhouse. It can be used in many different body products to create a soothing effect and even help with healing skin. Remember that regular honey from the store doesn't contain all the antioxidants that raw honey (unprocessed honey) does, so be sure to look for raw if you are planning on using honey for any of its healing qualities.

SOOTHE A COUGH. I remember my grandpa using this remedy many years ago. Simply have the patient swallow a spoonful of honey. To make an even better cough and cold remedy, mix the spoonful of honey into a mug of warm lemon water.

KICK-START HEALING CUTS. I love our homemade Healing Salve (page 69), but in a pinch, simply smear a bit of raw honey over a wound to help speed along the healing process.

ADD SOME EXTRA CONDITIONING TO YOUR CONDITIONER. When you make your homemade Conditioner (page 36), add a bit of honey for even more conditioning.

SOAK IN A SOOTHING BATH. Add a bit of honey in your bathwater or with your homemade Bath Salts (pages 43–44) to create some extra healing power for dry and cracked skin when taking a bath.

SWEETEN YOUR SALAD. Create a simple fruit salad with your favorite fruits (cantaloupe, grapes, and nectarines are yummy!) and a bit of honey. Chop the fruits, drizzle with a bit of honey, and serve.

REPLACE SUGAR IN CANNING AND PRESERVING RECIPES. Instead of making a sugar syrup for canning your fruits in, mix ¼ cup honey with 2½ cups filtered water for a honey syrup to cover them in.

MAKE SOME HONEY BUTTER. Honey butter is a fun special topping for biscuits, corn bread, and other treats. Whip 2 tablespoons honey with 1 stick (½ cup) softened butter. You can also add a pinch of ground cinnamon if you wish. For dairy-free honey butter, soften ½ cup coconut butter and whip with 2 tablespoons honey.

MAKE SOFTER BREADS. Replace the sugar and part of the liquid in a sweet quick bread recipe with honey for a softer bread.

HEALING LIP BALM. Add 1 teaspoon honey into my recipe for homemade Lip Balm (page 31) for a soft, healing lip balm with a hint of sweetness.

5 Uses for Plastic Bags

We don't make frequent trips to the grocery store, since we prefer to buy our food in bulk from a co-op, but somehow we still end up with a large number of plastic bags at our home. I always seem to find some use for them, though, so we tuck them away in the pantry until needed. Here are a couple of ways we've reused our plastic bags.

SMALL TRASH CAN BAGS. I keep a small trash can in our bedroom and in the bathroom so we have one on each level. The old storage crocks I use are the perfect size to fit a plastic bag inside. And how can you say no to free trash bags? In the last several years I don't think we've had to pay for little trash bags once.

TEMPORARY GAP FILLER. While working around the house we had some issues with gaps around pipes or in floors. For a temporary filling we simply stuffed plastic bags around the pipes (or occasionally in the opening of the pipe, depending on what work was going on) to stop air from coming through.

MINI GARDEN TARPS. During the days when garden plants are small and fragile, I've used plastic bags as a little tarp to cover the tops of the plants during a windstorm or light hailstorm. When our plants are small, we place cedar shingles around them as a little protective windbreak so the plastic bags fit right over the top of the shingles and sit snugly in place to protect the plants.

PILLOW STUFFING. While I would rather not sleep on a pillow stuffed with plastic bags, a dog or cat doesn't mind at all. Make a simple pet bed by sewing two blocks of fabric together in a rectangle and stuff the bed with old plastic bags. Just make sure to line-dry it instead of drying it in the machine.

CLEAN SHOE TRANSPORT. Many times when we are traveling or not at home, a pair of shoes gets wet or sandy or just plain dirty. I try to always carry plastic bags in the glove compartment of the car to put dirty boots or shoes in and transport them home.

5 Uses for Milk Jugs

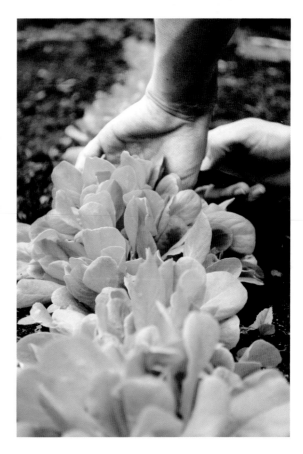

Have some extra milk jugs lying around? There are many uses for them, so make sure not to toss them! Here are five great ideas for your old milk jugs.

CREATE MINI GREENHOUSES. This is something that we've done in my family for many years. Through the winter, save up as many milk jugs as possible and cut the bottoms off. Use as a mini greenhouse over your newly started garden plants. Bury the bottom of the jug into the soil as far as possible and make sure to leave the cap off.

WATERING JUGS. I have an old jug that I use to fill my water filter on a daily basis. It's great for hauling a large amount of water easily from the sink to where I need to go!

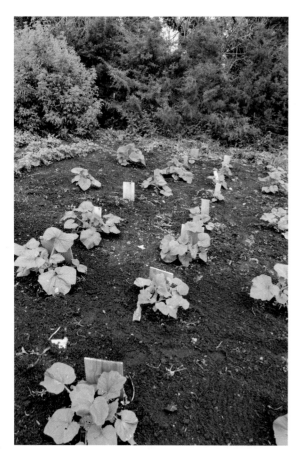

You can use your watering jug to water plants and flowers or anything you need to.

USE AS A SCOOP. Cut off a section of the flat front part of the milk jug container so you have a scoop, using the original handle of the jug as the handle of the scoop. This is great for scooping large bulk items or animal feed.

MAKE A CLOTHESPIN HOLDER. Cut open the front of the milk jug like you would to make a scoop and also cut out a small part of the handle so you can slip it over your clothesline. Place your clothespins inside the jug.

STORE AND POUR BIRDSEED. Birdseed can be hard to pour into birdfeeders if you buy it in a large bag. Use a funnel to pour the birdseed into an empty milk jug and use the jug to easily add the birdseed into your feeders.

7 Uses for Peppermint Essential Oil

Peppermint essential oil is one of the oils that I always have on hand. It's excellent for its invigorating scent in many home and body products, but it also has many helpful household uses.

KEEP SPIDERS AWAY. A bit of peppermint oil placed on cotton balls at strategic places around your house (windowsills, doorways, etc.) will help keep the spiders from coming in. If you have little ones and don't want to leave cotton balls lying around, simply use the cotton to apply a line of peppermint oil around windows, doors, or any other openings. Reapply as needed. This can also help with mice.

REMOVE TICKS. Place a drop of peppermint oil on the tip of a cotton swab and rub around the head of an embedded tick to help remove the tick.

RELIEVE A HEADACHE. Help to relieve your headache by mixing a drop or two of peppermint essential oil with a carrier oil (coconut oil, almond oil, jojoba oil, etc.). Rub on your neck or on your temples to help soothe and relieve a headache.

SOOTHE MOTION SICKNESS. Using the oil in the same way as described above (mixing a drop or two with a carrier oil), rub onto the insides of your wrists to help with motion sickness.

HELP FOR DANDRUFF. Adding a few drops of peppermint essential oil into your homemade Shampoo (page 35) will help fight dandruff. Tea tree oil will help with this as well.

INVIGORATE YOUR CLEANERS. Add peppermint essential oil into any of your homemade cleaner recipes to add a bit of an invigorating scent around your home as you clean.

STOP ANTS IN THEIR TRACKS. When you first see an ant or two in your home, place a bit of peppermint essential oil on a cotton ball and wipe over his tracks. The first ants are the "scouts" and if you allow them to form a path, they will tell the other ants where the food is. Peppermint essential oil can be your first line of defense if you see this happening.

11 Uses for Apple Cider Vinegar

Apple cider vinegar is one of those items that you can keep in your pantry for random uses around the house, just like baking soda. It's great in certain dishes and salad dressings, but it also has many other practical uses. Make sure to look for apple cider vinegar that has "the mother" and not one that has been filtered. The mother contains all the original healthy enzymes from the vinegar.

REMOVE WARTS. Place a cotton ball soaked in apple cider vinegar on a wart and hold it in place with a bandage or first aid tape. Leave in place for several hours and repeat as needed until the wart is gone.

KEEP YOUR CHICKENS (AND OTHER PETS) HEALTHY. Add a very small amount of apple cider vinegar to your chickens' (or other pets') water now and then to help maintain healthy birds. When we have used this remedy on our chickens, they always have the nicest, shiniest feathers.

QUICK AFTERSHAVE. Men who have trouble with stinging skin after shaving can dab on a bit of apple cider vinegar after a shave to stop the burning. Follow the vinegar with some aloe vera gel or homemade Aftershave Lotion (page 55).

MIX UP A RELISH. Make a quick relish with fresh produce and apple cider vinegar! Toss together some diced cucumber, diced onion, and diced apple plus a dash of apple cider vinegar, a bit of honey, a sprinkle of garlic, and some fresh dill. Mix all the ingredients for a fresh relish to serve with meals or sandwiches.

FRUIT FLY TRAP. Pour a small amount of apple cider vinegar in a glass or small container (jelly jars work great). Cover the top of the jar with plastic wrap and poke a few tiny holes in it. The fruit flies will be able to get in but not out! Place near fresh fruit in your kitchen.

SORE THROAT RELIEF. This is one of the worst-tasting solutions for a sore throat, so if you have an upset stomach with a sore throat you won't want to try this, but it does actually work very very well! Simply gargle with a bit of apple cider vinegar a few times daily as needed to help soothe a sore throat.

HEAL BRUISES FASTER. Soak up apple cider vinegar on a cool damp towel and use as a compress over a bruise to help it heal more quickly.

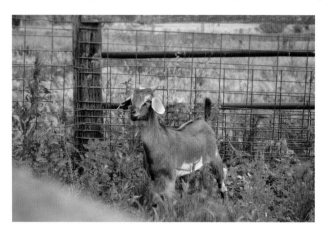

MAKE BUTTERMILK WHEN YOU NEED IT. If a recipe calls for buttermilk and you don't have any, you can make some quickly with apple cider vinegar! For every cup of buttermilk needed in a recipe, mix 1 cup whole milk with 2 teaspoons apple cider vinegar. Stir the mixture and let it stand for a few minutes so the milk can sour, then use as buttermilk in your recipe.

MAKE A QUICK SALAD DRESSING. I love to mix up this recipe when I don't have a dressing on hand but I want a fresh garden salad! In a pint or quart jar, mix 1 cup vegetable oil, ¼ cup apple cider vinegar, ¼ teaspoon paprika, and 1 teaspoon garlic salt. Place a lid on the jar and shake the mixture until combined. Shake before using and drizzle over salad as desired.

REMOVE NAIL FUNGUS. If you are suffering from some kind of nail fungus on your fingernails or toenails, soak them in straight apple cider vinegar as needed until the fungus goes away.

KITTY-STAY-AWAY SPRAY. If you are having trouble with a cat urinating in an area that you would rather it didn't, make a spray by simply adding full-strength apple cider vinegar to a spray bottle and spritzing it anywhere that you are having trouble. Reapply as needed.

5 Uses for Coffee Grounds

Coffee grounds are one of those wonderful things that seem like they are just trash but they are actually incredibly useful, especially once the coffee has been brewed! After your morning cup, instead of tossing them in the trash, make sure to save the grounds in a sealed jar or use them right away on one of these projects.

COFFEE-SCENTED CANDLES. The next time you make candles, toss a few scoops of old coffee grounds into the wax while it's melted. No need for artificial fragrances when you can scent your candles naturally!

CREATE A FUN ANTIQUE-LOOKING PAPER. Take some old coffee grounds and place them in a large casserole dish and add water. Dip a piece of paper into the mixture for a minute, then remove and let dry. Brush off any excess grounds once the paper is dry. You could also use this dye for fabrics or anything else you care to dye an antique color.

IN THE GARDEN. If your garden needs a dose of acid, add some old coffee grounds to the soil. Make sure you only add a small amount at a time to balance the soil. Blueberries especially love an acidic soil so make sure to add plenty of old coffee grounds around your blueberry plants.

ODOR ABSORBER. Place a small amount of old coffee grounds in a container and set it in the back of your fridge to help neutralize odors (baking soda works the same). You can also place coffee grounds (dry them out first) in the bottom of a trash can for the same purpose.

PEST DETERRENT. Sprinkle coffee grounds in ant mounds or around places cockroaches might go. Coffee grounds will also work as a deterrent for cats, so you can sprinkle them anywhere you don't want your kitty to be outside.

6 Uses for Beeswax

I love beeswax for all things body and beauty, but it has many great household uses as well. With everything from fixing squeaky doors to making homemade crayons, this list will inspire you and help you use any extra beeswax you might have around your home.

KEEP DOORS AND WINDOWS OPENING LIKE THEY SHOULD. Place a bit of softened beeswax in the joints and around the sides of windows to keep them opening and closing properly, easily, and without being squeaky. This also works on kitchen drawers that don't want to open.

RECONDITION WOODEN CUTTING BOARDS. Mix 1 teaspoon melted beeswax with 1 cup melted coconut oil. Rub on wooden cutting boards to recondition them and make them look brand-new again.

MAKE YOUR OWN CRAYONS. Create your own crayons for your little ones by melting 1 cup beeswax with 1 cup grated glycerin bar soap. Add a coloring agent of your choice (natural colored powders work best), pour into a mold (mini muffin tins or fun silicone molds work well) greased with oil, and let the crayons harden.

PRESERVE YOUR GARDEN TOOLS. Rub a bit of softened beeswax around the bases and handles of your garden tools to prevent rust and to keep them lasting longer.

WATERPROOF YOUR SHOES. Rub beeswax all over the surface of your shoes. Use a blow-dryer to melt the wax and then let the shoes rest for about 5 to 10 minutes until the beeswax has set into the shoes. This works best with canvas shoes.

MAKE YOUR OWN BEESWAX MODELING CLAY. Here's another fun project to make with your little ones. Melt ½ pound beeswax with 2 teaspoons lanolin and 2 tablespoons vegetable oil. (You may need to add a little more oil if your beeswax is crumbly.) Cool the mixture and then begin to mold it in your hands. The warmth of your body heat will create a moldable clay that your little ones can shape into whatever they want! You can also add natural coloring if desired.

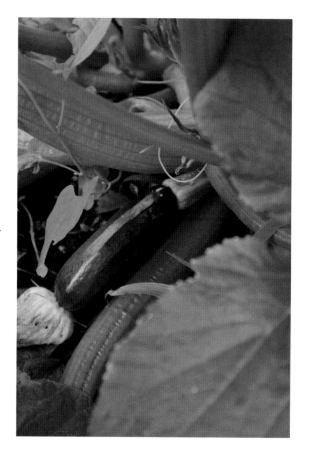

5 Uses for Shea Butter

Shea butter is another wonderful product that can be used for so many different body and beauty recipes. We use ours most often in everything from body lotion to diaper rash cream. Here are five more uses for shea butter that you'll want to try.

HEAL YOUR CRACKED HEELS. Shea butter can be a quick remedy for cracked heels. Rub gently into the affected heels (or fingers!) and reapply as needed.

STOP BUG BITES FROM ITCHING. If you are plagued by mosquito or other bug bites and you want some immediate relief, place a dab of shea butter over the affected area. (Coconut oil works as well.)

HELP RELAX LITTLE ONES FOR SLEEP. The secret to getting little ones to sleep more easily is to get them relaxed! You can make a quick foot rub for them with 1 tablespoon shea butter, 1 teaspoon coconut oil, and a few drops of lavender essential oil. Mix all the ingredients together and use as a foot rub when you are ready to help them wind down from the day.

SOOTHE MINOR BURNS. If you receive a burn and don't have any homemade Burn Salve (page 70) on hand, dab some shea butter over the affected area to help relieve the burn instantly.

RESTORE HAIR AND HELP WITH DRY SCALP. When you are making your homemade Shampoo (page 35), melt a little shea butter and add it in to help restore dry or brittle hair and soothe dry scalp.

12 Uses for Coconut Oil

Coconut oil seems to have an infinite amount of uses. In our little house we always keep a generous supply on hand and use it for everything from baking to putting in our homemade body products. Besides all of the amazing recipes in this book that use coconut oil, here are even more incredible uses.

REPLACE DAIRY IN MANY RECIPES. We've successfully replaced butter/milk/shortening with coconut oil in many different recipes. If you prefer not to have coconut flavor in what you are baking, use the expeller-pressed version.

REMOVE STICKINESS. Use coconut oil to remove gum or stickiness left from a label or sticker. For extra removal power, add some lemon essential oil to the coconut oil.

CONDITION YOUR WOODEN UTENSILS. If you love using wooden utensils, you will also love using coconut oil to keep them conditioned and lasting longer. Simply rub the oil over the clean utensils, bowls, or other wooden kitchenware.

KEEP YOUR PETS HEALTHY. Put a bit of coconut oil in your dog's food or on your kitty's fur so she licks it in. Coconut oil will help prevent hairballs, keep your pets' fur nice and shiny, and help with their overall health.

SOOTHE WINTER AND WIND CHAFING. If the wind and cold have gotten the best of you, rub a little coconut oil on the affected skin to soothe any chafing they may have caused.

STOP BABY'S CRADLE CAP. Use a soft facial exfoliating brush and rub coconut oil into baby's scalp in a circular motion. Rinse off the oil and repeat at bath time as needed until the cradle cap has gone away. Rubbing the scalp in a circular motion will also help with baby's hair growth.

TAME FRIZZY HUMIDITY HAIR. Place a very small amount of coconut oil on your fingertips and run through the ends of your hair on days when it's looking a bit frizzy. Avoid using too much or your hair will look greasy.

ADD TO SMOOTHIES. Add a spoonful of coconut oil into your smoothies for the health benefits and to help aid in digestion. Even if your family doesn't like to eat coconut oil, they may take it this way, as they shouldn't even be able to taste it.

SIMPLE FACIAL MOISTURIZER. When my skin is especially dry I like to use an extra moisturizer before I go to bed. First, dampen your face slightly with a wet towel and then rub in coconut oil. Dab ever so slightly with a dry towel (just to remove excess oil). Do this right before bed so you sleep with the oil on your face all night.

EASY DRY-SKIN-SOOTHING BATH. Add a spoonful of coconut oil into your bathwater and take a soak. The coconut oil will help to soothe and soften dry, irritated, and itchy skin. Make sure to keep hair out of the bath or it will become greasy.

RELIEF FOR FLY BITES. During the summer and fall we have lots of flies around the barn and the house. Placing a dab of coconut oil on the fly bites helps soothe them and take away the sting. You can do this for fly bites on animals as well.

USE AS A QUICK SHAVING CREAM. If you don't have time to make up our soothing recipe for homemade Shaving Cream (page 49), use a little coconut oil on your body while shaving to help the razor glide along. Just be careful, as it will make the shower slippery.

5 Uses for Witch Hazel

Witch hazel may seem like an odd thing to have in your home, but for many recipes it's a great, non-drying alternative to rubbing alcohol. In addition to our Non-Drying Hand Sanitizer (page 27), here are some other ways it can be used.

BRING DOWN PUFFINESS AROUND EYES. Just because you've had a few sleepless nights doesn't mean you need to look like you did. Place a bit of witch hazel in the fridge and then soak it up on a clean towel. Hold under your eyes to help reduce puffiness.

STOP BLEEDING. When used over fresh wounds, witch hazel can help to stop bleeding before you bandage up the wound. It will also help to disinfect the wound.

SOOTHE FRESHLY SHAVED SKIN. Like apple cider vinegar, witch hazel helps soothe freshly shaved skin and keeps it from becoming inflamed. It will also help to stop bleeding from any nicks from shaving.

STREAK-FREE SHINE. If you are having trouble with streaks on your glass and windows from your homemade Window Cleaner (page 104), add a bit of witch hazel to the mixture to help create a streak-free shine.

CLEAN YOUR JEWELRY. For a quick and easy jewelry cleaner, soak your dirty pieces of jewelry in a small container or bowl of pure witch hazel for about 20 minutes. Scrub the pieces with an old toothbrush and let them dry.

5 Uses for Epsom Salts

Epsom salts are something I always keep on hand at our house, because there are so many different things that we use them for, almost on a daily basis! If you bought Epsom salts for a project but weren't sure what to do with the rest of them . . . this list will help you get inspired!

DETOXIFYING FOOT BATH. Clean environmental toxins from your system by creating a simple foot bath. In a shallow container, fill up with several inches of very warm water. Add ¼ cup Epsom salts, ¼ cup baking soda, and 1 teaspoon bentonite clay powder (optional). Soak your feet until the water becomes cold. Make sure to drink plenty of water during your foot bath, to encourage draining.

GIVE YOUR GARDEN PLANTS A TREAT. Create a spray by dissolving ¼ cup Epsom salts in 1 gallon water. Pour the mixture into a spray bottle and spray your plants or simply pour it around them to add extra magnesium into the soil. This mix works especially well for tomato plants.

SOOTHE A SUNBURN. Add 1 cup Epsom salts to a warm bath and soak away the pain of a sunburn. For extra soothing power, add a dash of apple cider vinegar and/or coconut oil to the bath.

CREATE A QUICK SHOWER SCRUB. If your shower is looking a little dingy, mix ¼ cup Epsom salts with ¼ cup dish soap and use a sponge to scrub into your tub and shower walls. Rinse off the mixture when you are finished cleaning.

RELIEVE CRAMPED HANDS. We all know that Epsom salts can work wonders for inflammation, but they work particularly well for sore hands that may be inflamed from writing, typing, or other work. Fill up your bathroom sink with water and add ½ cup Epsom salts. Soak sore hands for 10 minutes to help bring down the inflammation. Use a thin lotion afterward (or even straight coconut oil) to help your hands retain moisture.

5 Uses for Sugar

We use sugar in many of our body scrubs, as well as in baking, of course. But that sweet sugar can do so much more. Since it's something I always have on hand, it's easy to add to various recipes and use for things around the house. Here are more ideas to get your creative juices flowing!

REFRESH A WASP TRAP. Boil 1 part water and 2 parts sugar together to make a sweet, semisticky syrup. Replace the store-bought liquids in your wasp traps or place in an old plastic bottle with a neck so that when the wasps fly in they can't fly back out.

MAKE SWEET SUN TEA. I prefer unsweetened sun tea, but my husband loves the sweet tea. To make a batch for my honey, I simply fill an old gallon jug with warm filtered water, 3 to 4 tea bags, and about ½ cup sugar. Shake this mixture in the jug and place it in the sun for several hours, swishing the mixture occasionally so the sugar dissolves. After a few hours, or when it's as dark as you like it, place the tea in the fridge. Serve cold.

MAKE YOUR KITCHEN SMELL BETTER. In a saucepan, boil a mixture of sugar and water to help absorb kitchen odors.

REMOVE GRASS STAINS. Take the article of clothing with a grass stain and soak the stained area with water until saturated. Sprinkle sugar over the top of the stain and let the garment sit for about an hour. Brush off the sugar and place the clothing in the washer and wash as normal.

MAKE A LIP SCRUB. Keep your lips soft by mixing up a simple lip scrub. In a small bowl, mix together 2 teaspoons sugar, ½ teaspoon coconut oil, and ½ teaspoon honey. Gently scrub onto lips and then rinse off or wipe off with a damp cloth.

8 Uses for Tea Tree Essential Oil

Tea tree essential oil is one of the staple essential oils that I recommend keeping around at all times. It has so many uses in body products because it's a natural antiseptic and antifungal. With tea tree and all other essential oils, keep in mind that they should not be used on infants and should be tested on a small area of skin first (and always applied with a carrier oil). Besides the recipes listed in this book, here are eight more uses for tea tree essential oil.

KEEP YOUR DIAPER PAIL FRESH. Diaper pails can be the worst offenders for smells. Sprinkle a few drops of tea tree essential oil in the bottom of your diaper pail to keep it clean and fresh.

PREVENT LICE. Add a few drops of tea tree essential oil to your homemade Shampoo (page 35) to help prevent lice.

BUMP UP THE POWER OF YOUR HOMEMADE CLEANERS. Add a few drops of tea tree essential oil into any of your homemade cleaners to add a special boost of cleaning power.

RESOLVE RINGWORM. Many don't realize that ringworm isn't a parasite, it's a fungus. To help treat ringworm, mix several drops of tea tree oil with a carrier oil (such as coconut oil, olive oil, etc.) and rub over a spot of ringworm. Repeat several times daily as needed.

CLEAR UP A NAIL FUNGUS. If you are suffering from a nail fungus, make a mixture similar to the one above (several drops of tea tree essential oil with a carrier oil) and rub into and around the affected nails several times a day until it has resolved.

CLEAR UP ACNE. If you have more acne than can be treated with the Zit Zapper Sticks (page 61), try adding a few drops of tea tree oil into your facial moisturizer or lotion to help clear up your entire face.

HELP WITH DANDRUFF. Add a few drops of tea tree essential oil into your homemade Shampoo (page 35) to combat dandruff and soap buildup on your scalp.

BRING DOWN A BOIL. Mix a few drops of tea tree essential oil with a carrier oil and dab on any boils on your skin several times a day until they clear up.

5 Uses for Lavender Essential Oil

If you are new to using essential oils, lavender oil should be one of the first ones on your list to buy. Lavender essential oil is antifungal and anti-inflammatory and can be used as an antiseptic. It also has a very calming scent that makes it perfect for those trying to relax. Besides the many recipes within this book that use lavender essential oil, here are a few other things that you can do with it.

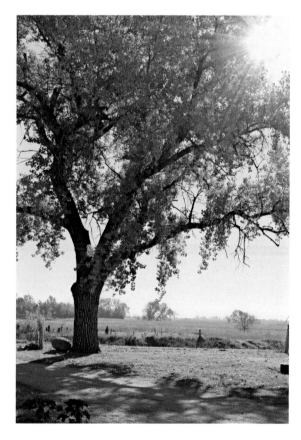

Note: Lavender essential oil should not be used by pregnant women.

HEAL BRUISES FASTER. Mix a few drops of lavender essential oil with a carrier oil (olive oil, coconut oil, etc.) and rub gently over a bruise to help promote blood flow so it will heal faster.

REPEL MOTHS. Place a bit of lavender essential oil on cotton balls and place in areas where moths have been a problem.

CALM DOWN. Add a few drops of lavender essential oil into any of your homemade lotions or bath products to create a calming and relaxing effect. Great for relieving anxiety or stress.

HELP WITH DANDRUFF. Just like tea tree essential oil, lavender essential oil can help with dandruff, so if you prefer the scent of lavender, use it instead. Just add a few drops into your homemade Shampoo (page 35).

ADDITIONAL HELP HEALING BURNS. Add a few drops of lavender essential oil into your homemade Burn Salve (page 70) to further promote healing.

5 Uses for Plaster of Paris

Plaster of Paris is a fun thing to have on hand when you have little ones because it has some great craft uses. Here are a couple of activities to try along with Rainbow Sidewalk Chalk (page 145).

STEPPING-STONES. Create a mold by cutting the bottom of an old plastic ice cream pail or small bucket. Mix the plaster of Paris according to the instructions on the box. Let it dry out slightly and then let your little ones place handprints, beads, stones, or their names into the plaster. Let it dry completely before popping it out of the mold and using it in the garden.

CHALK PAINT. Place ¼ cup plaster of Paris in a jar or small container with ½ cup water. Mix in a bit of washable paint or food coloring to color your paint and then let your little one use a paintbrush to paint it onto the sidewalk. Chalk paint will wash off the concrete just like sidewalk chalk.

MAKE LEAVES TO PAINT. Mix up the plaster of Paris according to the instructions on the box. Paint the plaster over thick leaves (and make sure the layer of plaster is thick) and let them dry undisturbed. Once dry, peel off the leaves and let your little ones paint them with pretty colors for décor.

MAKE A FOOTPRINT MEMORY. For this project you will need some sand and plaster of Paris. If you don't live near a beach, sand in the sandbox will work just fine. Mix up the plaster according to the instructions on the box. Have your little ones place their feet in the sand and push down until their footprints are still there when they remove their feet. Pour the plaster in the footprints and let it set until it's dry. Remove the plaster and file down any extra so you are just left with the cast footprints.

MAKE LARGE BEADS. Grab an ice cube tray or another small mold plus some plastic straws for this project. Mix the plaster of Paris according to the directions on the package. Add a little food coloring or paint to add color (or you can paint the beads later). Pour the plaster into the tray. Cut the straws into small pieces and place in the middle of each bead while the plaster is still a liquid to form the center hole. Let the beads dry and pop them out of the tray when they are finished. Remove the straws from the centers and you have beads!

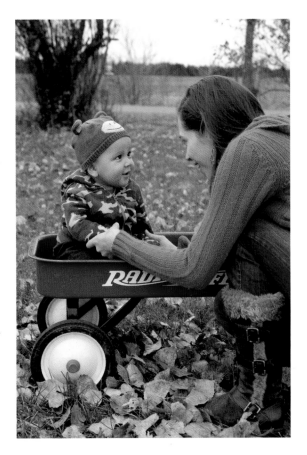

9 Uses for Olive Oil

Olive oil is another one of those items that I keep on hand at all times in my kitchen pantry. We generally use it for everything from baking and cooking to creating Olive Oil Candles (page 122). Here are even more things we use it for.

SHAVING CREAM IN A PINCH. If you are all out of shaving cream, you can use olive oil instead. Wipe over damp skin and shave as usual. Rinse off when finished. Keep in mind that your tub or sink may be slippery afterward.

KEEP YOUR MEASURING CUPS CLEAN. Do you have a hard time getting supersticky items like honey out of your measuring cups? Use your finger to coat the measuring cup first with some olive oil and then scoop or pour in what you need to measure. It will come out easily and cleanup will be a breeze.

GET A ZIPPER GOING AGAIN. If you have a zipper on a garment that seems to be locked into place, put a little olive oil around the zipper to get it going again.

HELP DRY SCALP. Add a bit of olive oil into your homemade Shampoo (page 35) or Conditioner (page 36) to help keep your scalp moisturized.

MAKE A SUPERQUICK SCRUB. If you want to make and use a sugar scrub but don't have much time, simply combine a little olive oil with ¼ cup sugar until it becomes the right consistency for a scrub and apply as needed. Rinse off when you are finished.

REPLACE BUTTER IN RECIPES. Many times you can make a recipe dairy-free by simply replacing the butter with olive oil.

QUICK AND SIMPLE SALAD DRESSING. In a blender, combine ¼ cup vinegar or lemon juice with 1 teaspoon garlic salt, ½ cup olive oil, and a dash of pepper. Blend until combined and use on your favorite salads.

REMOVE SAP FROM YOUR SKIN. Dab some olive oil on the sticky sap on your skin and rub until the sap is removed. Rinse clean.

MAKE A QUICK LUNCH. In a small saucepan, mix ½ cup olive oil with a few cloves of peeled, diced garlic. Simmer until the garlic begins to turn brown. Remove from heat and mix in a bit of pepper and salt and toss over cooked pasta.

7 Uses for Dish Soap

Dish soap, either homemade or store-bought, isn't just for keeping your dishes clean. It can also be used for a myriad of other purposes around your home. Here are a few ideas.

FLY SPRAY FOR PETS AND LIVESTOCK. In a spray bottle mix ¼ cup vinegar, 2 tablespoons dish soap, and 20 drops eucalyptus essential oil. Fill up the rest of the way with water. Spray on pets and livestock for flies and biting flies as needed.

Note: Not for use on cats.

GET RID OF ANTS. If you've found anthills and want to remove ants from your property, mix 1 cup dish soap with 1 cup vinegar and pour into the hill.

CLEAN AND SHARPEN BLENDER BLADES. In your blender place some water, a few ice cubes, and a little bit of dish soap. Pulse the mixture for a few minutes to clean and sharpen the blades. Rinse out the blender when finished.

USE AS A STAIN REMOVER. In a pinch, place pure dish soap over a stain if you aren't going to get a chance to wash it right away. Make sure you have a nice thick layer. Wash as normal.

CLEAN YOUR WALLS. Dish soap isn't just for cleaning dishes; you can clean all kinds of household surfaces with it! For walls, mix warm water with a bit of dish soap and wipe on to remove dirt and grime. Make sure to test on a small area first so you can be sure that it won't remove your paint.

KEEP BUGS OUT OF YOUR PLANTS. Even though a dish soap insecticide won't keep all the bugs out of your garden, it will help protect your plants. Mix some dish soap with water in a spray bottle and spritz on your plants as needed to keep some bugs away. This spray works best for worms and slugs.

MAKE A TILE SCRUB. Mix dish soap with a bit of sea salt to create a scrub for your tiles. Scrub onto tiles and wipe clean with a wet or damp cloth. Scrub into tile grout using an old toothbrush.

3 Uses for Vegetable Glycerin

Vegetable glycerin is one of the more unusual ingredients that I use in this book, but at our house it's a staple because we use it in those items so often! I like to buy it by the gallon to get a discount on it, so we always have plenty. Besides making homemade Outdoor Bubbles (page 147) and Diaper Rash Cream (page 138) with it, here are a few other things that I've used it for.

Note: Make sure you use food-grade vegetable glycerin for any project.

CREATE A THICK, DRY SKIN MASK. If you have a patch of very dry skin that you want to help, create a mixture of 2 tablespoons vegetable glycerin, 1 teaspoon honey, and

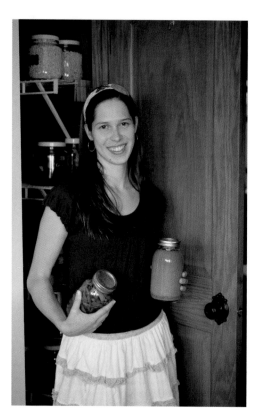

3 tablespoons uncooked old-fashioned oats. Mix together and spread over the dry skin. Let it sit for 15 to 20 minutes and then rinse off. Repeat as needed and follow with a thick moisturizing lotion.

CREATE AN ANTIFRIZZ POTION. Humidity doesn't do cute things to anyone's hair! Mix a bit of water with some glycerin, pick it up with your hands, and rub into your hair, particularly focusing on the ends of your hair after showering on a humid day.

MAKE FUN SNOW GLOBES. Grab a glass jar with a lid, water, glitter, vegetable glycerin, and anything else you want in the snow globe (we've used little beads, large shaped glitter, and more). Fill the jar three-quarters full with water and the rest of the way with glycerin and your glitter and add-ins. Secure the lid (you might want to use permanent glue if you have little ones) and shake the "globe" to watch the glitter fall slowly.

5 Uses for Bathroom Tissue Rolls

Bathroom tissue rolls . . . something every household has! The next time there is a finished bathroom tissue roll in your house, keep the center tube and try one of these projects with it.

TEACH LITTLE ONES SHAPES. Here's a fun activity that we did. Take the tissue roll center and bend one end into different shapes (square, heart, etc.). Let your little one dip the end of the roll in paint and use it as a stamp on construction paper.

MAKE A HEART CHAIN. Cut the empty bathroom tissue rolls so you have several ½-inch-wide sections. Shape into hearts and tie together to make cute decorative chains for a holiday or birthday.

MAKE A SIDEWALK CHALK MOLD. If you want to make some of my Rainbow Sidewalk Chalk (page 145) but don't have anything to use as a mold, place masking tape over one end of several empty bathroom tissue rolls. Then tape them together with the open ends facing up (tape them together so they are more stable as you pour in the chalk). Pour in the chalk recipe and let it set up. Once dry you can just peel the rolls away and remove your chalk. This chalk is large and easy to hold on to, perfect for little hands.

USE AS A VASE FILLER. If you are filling a vase with decorative items but don't want to buy a lot, place an empty bathroom tissue roll in the middle of the vase and fill the vase around the roll so it can no longer be seen. If you are worried about smaller items falling into the empty tissue roll, you can simply stuff it with old newspaper.

CREATE A SEEDLING STARTER. Cut empty bathroom tissue rolls in half and place upright in a large flat tube or container. Fill the rolls with dirt and place your seeds. Once you are ready to plant the seedlings outside, you can simply transplant the entire bathroom tissue roll—it will biodegrade into the soil as your seedling gets watered and grows.

5 Uses for Newspaper

In our previous home we had a woodstove for heat so all our old newspaper would always go to the stove for a fire starter. Now that we have a different heating system in our farmhouse, we use the newspaper for some other things once we've finished reading it. Here are some ideas that you can try for using your old newspapers.

CLEAN YOUR WINDOWS. This sounds a little crazy, but it really works! For a streak-free shine, spray glass cleaner on your windows and wipe dry with old newspaper. You can always use gloves if you don't want to get any ink on your hands, but it will leave your windows sparkling.

CLEAN UP A MESS. Continuing the trend I mentioned above, newspapers can be used in place of paper towels in many situations. Grab some old newspaper to clean up a liquid mess instead of a paper towel the next time you need one.

PREVENT ICE ON YOUR WINDSHIELD. We live in the land of cold and ice. If we plan to go somewhere on a cold winter day, the night before, we take newspaper and secure it with the windshield wiper blades over the windshield. When it's time to drive the car, there will be very little or no ice on the windshield to scrape off!

CATCH MUD FROM YOUR BOOTS. If you don't want to have to continually wash your rugs in the winter, place some old newspaper down where you come in the door as a place for boots and shoes that are wet and dirty. When the paper gets soaked, just change it out.

USE AS WRAPPING PAPER. Newspaper makes a very easy and non-see-through wrapping paper. Wrap up any gifts and tie with a pretty ribbon or bow to make them a bit fancy. All wrapping paper is going to be tossed in the trash anyway, so you might as well use something you already have!

5 Uses for Cornstarch

I love finding nonfood uses for the food in my pantry! The items that I can find many different uses for I often keep a large stock of because if I'm out of something else they can be substituted in a pinch. Cornstarch, potato starch, and arrowroot powder are all starches that I keep in my pantry regularly, and here are some great nonbaking uses for them! Where I say "cornstarch" in this section, potato starch and arrowroot powder work as well.

QUICK BABY POWDER. If you need a quick baby powder in a hurry and don't want to mix up the full recipe of homemade Baby Powder (page 142), you can use a sprinkle of cornstarch.

CREATE A SCENTED BODY POWDER. Place a few drops of your favorite essential oil in with some cornstarch and use as a scented body powder. It can also be placed in shoes as a fast odor absorber in a pinch.

STOP THE SQUEAKING. If you have a place in your floor or on a step that is particularly creaky, dust the area with some cornstarch and sweep it into the cracks.

CLEAN UP OIL AND GREASE STAINS. If you've spilled some oil or grease onto your floor or carpet, it can be hard to get out with just a damp rag. Sprinkle some cornstarch over the spot and let it sit for at least an hour. After that time you should be able to vacuum or wipe up the spot.

POLISH YOUR SILVER. You can shine up any silver dishes or silverware in your home with cornstarch. Just make a paste with the starch and water, buff the silverware until you've removed all the paste, and wipe off with a dry towel.

10 Uses for Oats

We all know that oats can make for a frugal and hearty breakfast, but did you also know that you can use either old-fashioned or quick-cooking oats for all sorts of homemade body products and home remedies? Here are 10 extra uses for the packages of grains sitting on your pantry shelf.

CREATE AN ANTI-ITCH POTION TO STOP THE STING OF POISON IVY. Either pour a cup or two of oats directly into your bathwater (tepid water, not hot), or mix the oats with a little bit of filtered water until it forms a paste that you can spread on the affected area. Leave the oats on your skin for at least 20 minutes or until the itching starts to subside.

CREATE A SOOTHING MILK BATH. If you have dry skin, an oatmeal milk bath is the perfect solution! Add 1 cup oats, 1 cup milk, and 1 tablespoon honey to your bath. Stir this around your tub and enjoy your soak. Add a bit of coconut oil for extra nourishment.

CREATE AN ACNE FACE MASK. In a blender, grind ½ cup oats until you create a fine powder. Pour into a small bowl and add 1 tablespoon baking soda. Slowly mix in filtered water until you make a paste. Spread evenly over your face (note: some skin can be sensitive to baking soda, so test on a small area of skin first) and let it sit for 3 to 5 minutes before washing off with water.

REINVIGORATE A DRY SCALP. Use the same mixture as the one for the acne face mask but don't add the water. Rub the dry mixture into your hair and rinse out in the shower to help cleanse a dry scalp. Finish your shampoo session with an apple cider vinegar rinse (page 36).

CREATE A FOOT SCRUB. In a small bowl, mix ½ cup oats with 2 tablespoons coconut oil and a few drops of peppermint essential oil. Rub on your feet to help smooth and refresh them after a long day. Wipe off with a damp towel.

STRETCH YOUR MEAT. Oats make a great ground beef stretcher because once you mix them into the meat, you won't even know that they are there! Add up to ¼ cup oats per pound of ground beef. Add to your meat for meat loaf, meatballs, and hamburgers, or even just add to ground beef that you are cooking for tacos, casseroles, etc.

ABSORB SMELLS AROUND THE HOUSE. Oats can be a great odor absorber. To use them in this way you will simply need to pour some into a dish or container and place in the offending area. To add a little fragrance to the area, mix a few drops of your favorite essential oil into the oats.

KEEP YOUR ENERGY UP. Use oats to make these quick and easy no-bake energy bites! Mix 1 cup uncooked old-fashioned oats, ½ cup nut butter (or sunflower seed or

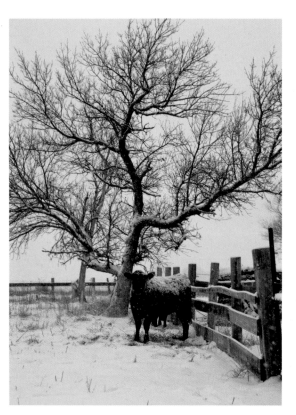

coconut butter for those with nut allergies), ¼ cup honey or maple syrup, 1 cup coconut flakes, and ¼ cup mini chocolate chips (optional). Mix all those ingredients together. Chill the dough for 30 minutes and then form into small balls. Enjoy immediately or store in the fridge for later.

USE AS A THICKENER. If you are out of cornstarch or another thickener that you planned on using in a soup, casserole, or similar dish, simply grind up a small amount of oats in the blender until it becomes a powder. Add to your dish just as you would another thickener.

MAKE A POWERFUL HAND SCRUB. In a small bowl, mix ½ cup oats with 3 tablespoons milk until it forms a thick paste. Use as a hand scrub to clean off grimy hands.

5 Uses for Clothespins

Clothespins are a fun thing to have around your home because it seems like they are always needed for some purpose or another . . . to hold things together, to close things, to hang things . . . so many uses for clothespins and so little time! Here are a few to try.

CHIP AND CRACKER BAG CLOSER. I always seem to need more clips to keep my bags of food closed so the humidity doesn't get in. Once I bought some fancy, colorful "chip clips" from the store and realized that I'd very much overpaid when I could have gotten 100 clothespins for the same price I paid for ten chip clips!

SUPPORT GROWING STEMS. In the garden we sometimes have trouble getting the new climbing plants to start climbing their trellis, but the solution is simple: clip the vine to the trellis with a clothespin so the vine will learn where it needs to go. Just make sure you get the vine in the hole of the clothespin or you will pinch it too tight.

TACK UP YOUR TO-DO LIST. Have a recipe you are making or a to-do list that you can't forget about? Use a clothespin to pin it somewhere that you will see it: a bathroom mirror, a stove range hood, or anywhere else with high visibility.

MAKE A MISSING SOCKS LAUNDRY LINE. String up a small laundry line in your wash room, if you have the space, and clip clothespins to it to hold the socks that are missing their partners.

HOLD YOUR TABLECLOTH IN PLACE. Use clothespins to clamp a tablecloth together under the table so it won't move out of place.

5 Uses for Lemons

Throughout this book, lemons are used in various dishes and skin care products, but they can be useful for much more than that! Here are five more uses for those sour little lemons.

PREVENT FRUITS FROM TURNING BROWN. Most browning on fruits and vegetables can be stopped with a bit of lemon juice. Just coat the food with a few drops of fresh lemon juice and it should last much longer.

MAKE A QUICK PRODUCE WASH. Like baking soda and vinegar, lemon juice can also be used as a produce wash since it has disinfectant qualities. Just squeeze fresh juice into a spray bottle and use as you would any other produce wash.

CREATE A DEODORIZER. Lemon peels make an excellent deodorizer. Instead of tossing them in the trash the next time you use a lemon, toss them in the bottom of the trash can or in the back of the fridge to create a pleasant scent and help deodorize unpleasant smells.

CLEAN OUT YOUR GARBAGE DISPOSAL. If you have a garbage disposal and it hasn't been smelling very nice, toss your old lemon peels in it along with a bit of ice. The ice will help sharpen the blades of your disposal and the lemon peels will leave it smelling fresh.

REMOVE SOAP BUILDUP. If you have any kind of soap buildup in your shower, on your appliances, or in other areas of your home, rub a little fresh lemon juice over the area and scrub lightly with a damp towel to help remove the grime.

5 Uses for Aloe Vera

I love keeping aloe vera gel on hand at all times and I even like to keep an aloe plant in my kitchen for fresh gel. We use aloe vera gel in several body and beauty recipes, but here are more uses for it. When looking for an aloe vera gel, make sure to buy one without added ingredients or dyes.

SOOTHE A RASH. Place a dab of aloe vera gel on bug bites or rashes to help soothe them and bring down the inflammation. Aloe vera can also take the sting out of allergic skin reactions.

SOFTEN ROUGH ELBOWS. If you get dry skin on your elbows in the winter, aloe vera gel can help! Mix together a scrub with ¼ cup aloe vera gel, ¼ cup sugar, and 1 tablespoon honey. Scrub gently over dry, rough elbows and follow with a soothing lotion. Use as often as needed.

USE AS A MOISTURIZER. If you are in need of a facial moisturizer that is oil-free, try aloe vera gel! It's great for hydrating and healing skin and won't be the cause of more breakouts like traditional moisturizer can be.

SPEED UP HAIR GROWTH. If your little one is having trouble getting hair back after having cradle cap, massage a little aloe vera gel into the baby's scalp during bath time to help hair grow back more quickly.

REPLACE AN ICE PACK. If you have a little one who refuses to hold an ice pack on a fresh bruise, keep a little aloe vera gel in the fridge. When they come to you with a new owie, just place a little of the cool gel on the hurt. The gel will soothe and cool the spot.

5 Uses for Ziplock Bags

I will admit that I have an issue with tossing plastic bags if they are hardly used. It's just money down the drain! Over the years we've found several ways to reuse those little ziplock bags around the home. We've found that the freezer bags are more worth reusing; the regular storage bags don't seem to hold up well to being repurposed.

HOLD YOUR TOILETRIES. Rinse out and dry an old ziplock bag and use it to store any toiletries that may leak on a trip that you are taking. We love doing this for camping trips because we can pack all the toiletries together, yet each person has their own individual little baggies with their items, so it's easy to separate them.

USE AS A DECORATING BAG. I don't do much decorating with frosting, so I've never owned a set of decorating bags and tips, but a repurposed ziplock bag works just as well. Place your frosting or whatever you are using into a bag, cut a tiny hole in one corner, and pipe your frosting just as you would with any decorating bag.

MAKE YOUR OWN ICE PACK. All you need is a sponge, a ziplock bag, and some rubbing alcohol. Soak the sponge in the alcohol and place in the ziplock bag. Seal the bag and place it in the freezer. The alcohol won't freeze but it will cool down, making it the perfect reusable ice pack!

MAKE SQUISHY SENSORY BAGS. My little ones love it when we make these! Using an old washed and dried ziplock freezer bag, fill it halfway with hair gel (I pick up

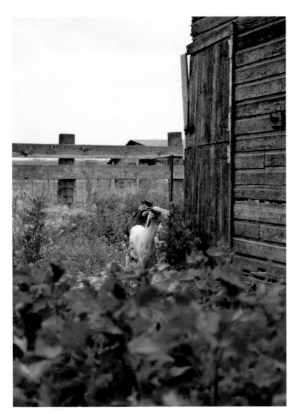

inexpensive gel at the dollar store). Add a bit of food coloring or other fun things (marbles, small toys, anything not sharp) and seal the bag. Use masking tape around the edges, stick the bag to your table, and let your little ones "draw" and squish the bag.

STORE GAMES AND PUZZLES. When we moved into our farmhouse we simply had no room for the huge stack of board games that we'd collected. I took all of the pieces from each game and placed them in their own gallon-size ziplock bags and put all the game boards in a stack. We store all the bags and boards in an old steamer trunk in our living room and they take up less than a quarter of the space that they did before!

5 Uses for Eggshells

Eggshells are something that no little hobby farm is ever without. Thankfully, the shells can be just as useful as the eggs! Here are just a few things that we've done with eggshells.

USE THE CALCIUM. Crush the shells and use for added calcium in your garden or even for your chickens! If feeding eggshells to your chickens, make sure they are completely dry and nothing remains of the whites and the yolk, or your chickens may start pecking at their own eggs.

USE AS A SCRUB OR PUMICE ALTERNATIVE. In household cleaner recipes for which you are looking for a little bit of scrubbing power (such as the All-Purpose and Window Cleaner, page 103), crush and powder some eggshells and add them to the recipe.

START YOUR SEEDLINGS. For plants that enjoy an extra boost of calcium and don't need to be large and established when placed outdoors, put a little bit of soil in the bottom of an eggshell and plant your seeds. Once the plant is an inch or two tall, transplant outside right into the ground, eggshell and all!

MAKE A SCRUBBER FOR POTS AND PANS. Crush the eggshells into a powder and use with your dish soap to scrub particularly dirty pots and pans. Make sure to wash separately from other dishes and to rinse off when you are done scrubbing; otherwise you might have some stuck-on eggshell crumbs.

MAKE MOSAIC ART. When I was little we used to dry out eggshells, crush them, and then use the pieces of the different-colored eggs for mosaic artwork. Just have some kind of heavy poster board for your young ones to glue the eggshells to and let them create!

5 Uses for Tea Bags

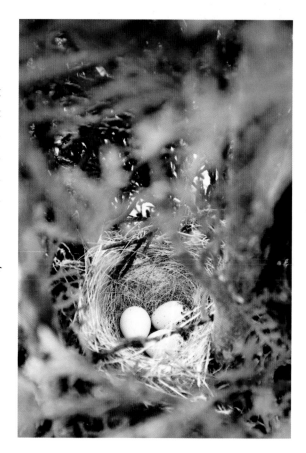

I don't know about you, but for me, tossing the tea bag after making tea has always felt somewhat wasteful. It just seems like there is so much in the bag still that I hate to get rid of it. Of course, just like most things around your home, you can give those tea bags a second life before they head to the trash! Here are a few ideas to get you started.

FURNITURE STAIN. If you have a bag of black tea, place the tea bag in a small amount of water and press on the tea leaves to get every last drop of tea from the bag. Once you've got a concentrated mixture, use it for staining scuffed up furniture or for antiquing furniture that you are painting or creating.

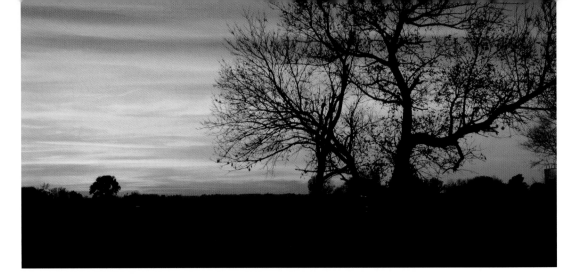

MAKE YOUR MEAT MORE SAVORY. If you have meat with little flavor or that is a little bit gamy, place a tea bag in with your marinating meat to boost the flavor.

USE AS A HAIR RINSE. If you prefer not to use the hair rinse described on page 36, you can also use tea to give your hair a rinse. It will help condition your hair, and if it's a dark tea and you have dark hair, it can even help boost your color and shine.

CREATE A DRAINAGE LAYER. If you have several used tea bags, place them at the bottom of a pot before planting to help hold moisture in the pot and release it as needed to your plants.

REDUCE KITTY LITTER SMELLS. Take a few used tea bags and open them up so the contents can dry out. Once dry, sprinkle the tea into your kitty's litter box to help reduce odors.

Index

sugar cookie mix, 213
See also baking mixes;
    pancake and waffle mix
grapefruit essential oil, 23
grapeseed oil, 23
grass stains, 278
grease and oil stains, 286–87
green tea facial wash, 62

H

hair care, 35–37
    conditioner, 36, 265
    cradle cap in babies,
      274–75, 291
    dandruff, 269, 279, 280
    detangling spray, 38
    dry scalp treatments, 46,
      274, 282, 287
    dry shampoo, 25–26, 142
    frizzy hair treatments, 275,
      284
    hair rinses, 36–37, 294
    hair spray, 45
    wet shampoos, 35,
      132–33, 269, 279
hamburger help mix, 167
handmade bread mix,
    224–25
hand sanitizer, non-drying,
    27
hand scrubs, 50–51, 288
hand soaps, foaming,
    53–54
hard water, 93, 94
headache relief, 269
healing. *See* first aid
healing hand scrub for
    gardeners, 50–51
herbs
    growing, 37, 238, 263

herbal infusions for
    shampoos and
    conditioners, 35–36,
    37
herb dip and spread mix,
    238
herbed garlic rice side dish
    mix, 176
herb seasoning mix, 241
Italian seasoning, 243
storing, 262
holiday spice foaming hand
    soap, 54
honey, 23, 80, 265–66
    honey butter, 172, 266
    substituting sugar for, 261
honey bun cake, 192
hot chocolate mix, 216
hot dogs, corndog bites, 229
household recipes, 83–125
    about, 84–85
    all-purpose cleaner, 103
    ant spray, 113–14
    basic ingredients, 11
    candles, 122–24
    carpet cleaner and
      shampoo, 105
    cleaning wipes, 101–2
    cooking spray, 87
    deodorizer disks, 121
    dish soaps, 88–89
    dishwasher detergent, 94
    dusting spray, 96–97
    fabric freshener spray, 111
    fabric softeners, 108–9
    floor cleaner, 100
    furniture polish, 98–99
    garden pest sprays,
      115–16, 283
    gel air fresheners, 118
    jewelry cleaners, 125, 276

    laundry detergent, 106
    oven cleaner, 92–93
    produce washes, 91, 290
    stain stick, 112
    wax melts, 124
    weed spray, 117
    window cleaner, 103–4,
      276
    wrinkle release spray, 110
housekeeping tips, 85–86,
    94, 99, 105, 181
    baking soda uses, 264,
      265
    beeswax uses, 272
    plastic bag uses, 266,
      267
    See also cleaning; kitchen
      tips; laundry and
      clothing; pests

I

ice packs, 291
icy windshields, preventing,
    286
ingredients
    for body care, beauty,
      and household recipes,
      10–15, 22–24, 261
    pantry staples, 163
    simple substitutions,
      260–61
    storage and containers, 13,
      14–15
    where to buy, 13
insects
    bites and stings, 264, 273,
      275, 290
    See also pests; *specific insects*
instant oatmeal packets,
    204–5

instant refried beans,
234–35
Italian dressing mix, 243
Italian seasoning, 243

J

jewelry cleaners, 125, 276
jojoba oil, 23

K

kitchen, recipes for, 87–94
   cooking spray, 87
   dish soaps, 88–89
   dishwasher detergent, 94
   oven cleaner, 92–93
   produce washes, 91, 290
   See also mixes, make-ahead
kitchen tips
   oiling measuring cups,
     281
   reconditioning cutting
     boards, 272
   See also cleaning

L

laundry and clothing,
   106–12
   clothing tips, 111, 112,
     133, 147
   fabric freshener spray,
     111
   fabric softeners, 108–9
   laundry detergent, 106
   milk jug clothespin holder,
     268
   missing socks line, 289
   moth repellent, 279
   shoe spray, 81

stain and spot removal, 72,
   112, 142, 278, 286–87
stain stick, 112
stuck zippers, 282
waterproofing shoes, 272
wrinkle release spray, 110
lavender essential oil, 23,
   279–80
lemon(s)
   freezing lemon juice, 45
   lemon juice facial wash,
     62
   lemon poppy seed body
     scrub, 73
   uses for, 289–90
lice, 278
lip balms, 31–32, 266
lip gloss, smooth and shiny,
   33–34
lip scrub, 278
litter boxes, 294
lotions
   aftershave lotion, 55, 270
   baby lotion, 137
   body butters, 76–77
   lotion bars or sticks,
     63–64
   refreshing peppermint foot
     lotion, 78
   simple sunblock lotion or
     bar, 56–57
   sunburn relief cream, 58
   whipped coconut oil
     lotion, 46–47

M

mango body butter, 77
mango butter, 23
meal planning
   about, 246–47

menus with recipes,
   249–55
meat
   adding tea to marinades,
     294
   beef stroganoff menu,
     254
   beef stroganoff mix, 168
   buying in bulk, 169
   chili mix, 179
   hamburger help mix, 167
   homemade sausage, 198
   roast menu, 249
   seasoning mixes, 240–41
men
   aftershave lotion, 55, 270
   aftershave skin soothers,
     270, 276
   body wash for, 40
menus, 249–55
mice, 111, 268
milk jug uses, 267–68
minty fresh face mask, 67
mixes, make-ahead,
   161–243
   about, 162–66
   baked oatmeal mix, 202–3
   baking mix, all-purpose,
     171–73
   beef stroganoff, 168
   bread mixes, basic, 223–25
   brownie mix, 182–85
   cake mixes, 186–92
   chai tea mix, 219
   chicken help, 169
   chicken noodle soup mix,
     178
   chili mix, 179
   chocolate chip cookie mix,
     209–10
   cobbler mix, 232–33

coffee creamer, powdered, 220–21
corn bread mix, 226–29
cream of soup mix, 181
dip mixes, 237–38
faux bouillon, 177
gluten-free flour mix, all-purpose, 164
hamburger help, 167
hot chocolate mix, 216
instant oatmeal packets, 204–5
instant refried beans, 234–35
meal planning with, 245–55
muffin mix, 199–201
onion soup mix, 180
pancake and waffle mix, 195–98
pet treat mixes, 157–59
pudding mixes, 206–8
quick bread mix, 230–31
rice side dish mixes, 174–76
seasoning mixes, 239–43
storing, 164
sugar cookie mixes, 211–15
modeling clay, beeswax, 273
moisturizers, 275, 290
moisturizing body wash, 39–40
See also lotions
mosaic art, 293
moth repellent, 279
motion sickness, 269
muffins
basic muffins, 199–201
corndog muffins, 229
muffin mix, 199

mushroom soup, cream of, 181

N

nail fungus, 271, 278
newspaper, 285–86
no-bake energy bites, 288
non-petroleum jelly, 28
lip gloss, 33–34

O

oats and oatmeal, 287–88
baked oatmeal, 202–3
baked oatmeal mix, 202
instant oatmeal packets, 204–5
no-bake energy bites, 288
oatmeal cookie body scrub, 75
oatmeal face masks, 67, 283–84, 287
oil and grease stains, 286–87
olive oil, 23, 281–82
olive oil candles, 122–23
onion(s)
onion aphid spray, 116
onion soup mix, 180
quick cucumber-onion-apple relish, 270
organic ingredients, 12–13
outdoor bubbles, 131, 147
oven apple pancake, 198
oven cleaner, 92–93

P

paints
chalk paint, 280

finger paints, 153
"painting" with water, 151
watercolor paints, 151
pancake and waffle mix, 195
basic pancakes or waffles, 196
coffee cake with crumble topping, 197–98
fried chicken, 197
oven apple pancake, 198
pancake supper menu, 252
pantry staples, 163
pasta
in beef stroganoff mix, 168
in chicken help mix, 169
chicken noodle soup, 178
in hamburger help mix, 167
Italian pasta salad, 243
quick pasta with olive oil and garlic, 282
in rice side dish mixes, 174–76
pears, brown sugar baked, 255
peppermint essential oil, 23, 58, 268–69
ant spray, 113–14
refreshing peppermint foot lotion, 78
pests, 114
ant repellents, 113–14, 229, 269, 272, 283
coffee grounds for, 272
fly spray for pets and livestock, 282
fruit fly trap, 270
garden pest sprays, 115–16, 283
lice, 278